Luciano Teixeira
Francisco Prado Reis
Cristiane Oliveira

Childhood Obesity in the Quilombola Community of Mussuca - Sergipe

Luciano Teixeira
Francisco Prado Reis
Cristiane Oliveira

Childhood Obesity in the Quilombola Community of Mussuca - Sergipe

Prevalence of overweight and obesity in children and adolescents from the Quilombola Community of Mussuca - Sergipe

ScienciaScripts

Imprint

Cover image: www.ingimage.com

This book is a translation from the original published under ISBN 978-620-2-17465-7.

Publisher:
Sciencia Scripts
is a trademark of
Dodo Books Indian Ocean Ltd. and OmniScriptum S.R.L publishing group

120 High Road, East Finchley, London, N2 9ED, United Kingdom
Str. Armeneasca 28/1, office 1, Chisinau MD-2012, Republic of Moldova, Europe
Printed at: see last page
ISBN: 978-620-7-41818-3

Table of contents:

DEDICATION

I dedicate this work to my beloved mother who has always led me along the paths of love, to my wonderful wife, Aline, who has always been by my side, supporting and encouraging me to face all the difficult moments, to my dear daughter Natália who has always been encouraging me. To my dear father - *in memoriam.* The love I feel for you is immeasurable!

ACKNOWLEDGMENTS

To God for the gift of life, for showing me that I am capable of overcoming all obstacles and coming out of the battle stronger and stronger.

To the Postgraduate Program in Health and Environment at Tiradentes University, for allowing me and my colleagues to walk the path of research and academic teaching.

To my mother for her love and dedication, for guiding me, always showing me that the road would not be easy, but that I should always keep going regardless of the obstacles. I know that she often gave up her dreams so that I could fulfill mine.

To my wife, for her patience, dedication, companionship and love.

My daughter, who is the greatest treasure in my life.

To my sisters and nephews whom I love so much, for their affection and deep love.

To my family, whom I love too much, the reason for my life. If I could choose a family, I would always choose you.

To Professor Dr.[3] Claudia Moura de Melo for her affection, advice and contributions to my education.

To Professor Dr. Cristiane Costa da Cunha Oliveira, for her contributions to enriching the work, especially for her help with the mobility project (PROMOB).

To my friends, the old ones who have been with me for a long time and the new ones.

To all the professors of the Postgraduate Program in Health and Environment. To my fellow master's students, for their conviviality, affection and friendship. To UNIT for the scholarship. Finally, to everyone who was with me at this stage of my life.

And finally to my advisor **Prof. Dr. Francisco Prado Reis**, thank you for the opportunity to learn from you, for your patience and dedication.

SUMMARY

Childhood obesity has been increasing rapidly over the last few decades, and this has been characterized as a true global epidemic. This fact is very worrying, because the association of obesity with metabolic alterations, such as hypertension and glucose intolerance, which are risk factors for type 2 diabetes mellitus and cardiovascular disease, until a few years ago was more evident in adults, but can now be observed in children and adolescents. Even with the political mobilization to organize the quilombola communities, there is a situation in which the indicators point to the continued social vulnerability of the communities and a certain distance between these populations and social policies and their benefits. Problems such as the poor quality of education, insufficient health and sanitation services and precarious housing are recurring demands in Sergipe's quilombola communities. Thus, we have a situation in which the recent achievements in terms of recognizing the rights of the remnants of quilombos have not led to significant improvements in the living conditions of these populations, nor have they succeeded in reducing the distance between social inequalities and the communities' surroundings. The aim of this study was to assess the prevalence of childhood overweight and obesity in groups of children aged between five and fourteen in the public school system of the Quilombola Community of Mussuca, in the municipality of Laranjeiras in the state of Sergipe, and to identify its main causes. In order to carry out this work, it was necessary to measure the height and weight of each child, and based on this data the BMI was calculated. Data on food consumption and physical activity were obtained through interviews using a specific form. This study assessed 301 schoolchildren aged between 5 and 14, 152 (50.5%) female and 149 (49.5%) male. It was concluded that the prevalence of overweight children and adolescents was 22.6% and that obesity accounted for 13.3% (40). Thus, for a reliability level of 5% and a sample size of 301 children and adolescents, the admitted error was 3.81%. The results suggest that food consumption plays an important role, but that a sedentary lifestyle can also contribute to excess weight in children and adolescents. Recognizing that the problem has a multi-causal origin should guide public policies aimed at this age group in the quilombola community in order to prevent this nutritional problem.

Key words: Anthropometry; Childhood obesity; Health of specific groups; Sedentary lifestyle.

Chapter 1

1 - INTRODUCTION

The majority of the Brazilian population is made up of black or brown people, and a significant proportion of this human contingent is still found today in the poorest strata of the population, a historical consequence of a series of inequities to which black people and their descendants have been subjected, including in relation to health care (PINTO, 2014).

In Brazil, the places occupied by black slaves who fled forced labor and resisted recapture by the slave forces became known as quilombos. After the abolition of slavery, many quilombos gave rise to today's quilombo communities. The members of these communities have strong cultural ties, maintaining their traditions, religious practices, relationship with working the land and system of social organization (CARVALHO, 1995).

The definition of traditional peoples and communities was established in Decree No. 6.040 of February 7, 2007, article 3, item I, which defines "... culturally differentiated groups who recognize themselves as such, who have their own forms of social organization, who occupy and use territories and natural resources as a condition for their cultural, social, religious, ancestral and economic reproduction, using knowledge, innovations and practices generated and transmitted by tradition..." (BRAZIL, 2007).

Although this understanding extends to black people in general (people of African descent, black people living in cities, individuals belonging to the remaining quilombo communities), when it comes to health care, special concern should be reserved for individuals belonging to the so-called quilombo communities (FREITAS, 2011).

Quilombola communities are holders of an invaluable historical and cultural heritage. They preserve centuries-old cultural practices, brought by their ancestors directly from the African continent, religiosity and art. The concept of quilombo and quilombola goes beyond a repository of memory and history. They are concrete subjects who need to be socially included in terms of their traditions (CORREIA; COSTA; BALBINO, 2007).

Ribeiro, (2015), considered that quilombola communities in Brazil experience problems in terms of food and nutrition, which may include disorders such as obesity in children and adolescents. This may make this study relevant.

According to the WHO, in 2008 there were approximately 1.5 billion overweight adults worldwide, around 200 million obese men and 300 million obese women and, in 2010, almost 43 million children were overweight (WHO, 2011).

Obesity in children and adolescents leads to orthopedic problems, sleep apnea, some types of cancer and psychological disorders, which can lead to death. It is important to emphasize that all these problems cause a poor quality of life and a cost to the public purse in terms of preventing, treating and recovering the health of obese individuals (PELLANDA. et al., 2002).

Studies in Brazilian quilombola communities have shown a picture of epidemiological transition, as they face food insecurity and can present significant rates of overweight and obesity, including in children (SOARES; BARRETO, 2014).

As this is a social segment with characteristics of economic disadvantage and social vulnerability, it is possible that systematized information on healthy eating and nutrition is not sufficiently accessible to prevent overweight and obesity in children and adolescents (GUIMARÁES; SILVA, 2015).

In view of the scarcity of studies on obesity in northeastern Brazil and in quilombola communities in Sergipe, and in order to understand how the Mussuca quilombola community in Laranjeiras - SE, one of the largest in the state, fits into this current context, in which more and more children and adolescents have become victims, this study was carried out.

Chapter 2
2 - OBJECTIVES

2.1. General Objective

- To determine the epidemiological profile of obesity and overweight in children and adolescents in the Quilombola community of Mussuca - Laranjeiras, SE.

2.2. Specific objectives

- To identify the percentage of obese children and adolescents between the ages of 5 and 14 in the quilombola community of Mussuca.
- To analyze the relationship between obesity and overweight among those surveyed according to socio-demographic variables, dietary habits and physical activity;

Chapter 3

3 . THEORETICAL FRAMEWORK

3.1.- Quilombolas - Vulnerable Populations

Quilombola communities are population groups that are remnants of former quilombos, representing the resistance of black Brazilians. They are located in various regions of the country, especially in rural areas, have a relative degree of geographical isolation and experience marked social and health inequalities (MONEGO et, al, 2010).

These communities carry a great deal of historical complexity because they are the result of resistance to the process of slavery imposed for centuries on black people, and even after the Golden Law they are still marginalized by society (SALLES, 2005).

Many quilombos, after the abolition of slavery, gave rise to today's quilombo communities. The members of these communities have strong cultural ties, maintaining their traditions, religious practices, relationship with working the land and system of social organization (CARVALHO, 1995).

From a legal point of view, quilombola communities were officially recognized by the Brazilian state in 1988, Article 68 of the Transitional Constitutional Provisions Act (BRASIL, 2002). This recognition, however, has not been enough to meet the needs of these groups, particularly among children, who are considered the most vulnerable, with high rates of nutritional deficits and little access to education and health services, showing the low effectiveness of the coverage of the programs proposed by governments aimed at social promotion (FERREIRA et al. 2011).

Specifically, from the point of view of health, we can see the process of nutritional and epidemiological transition shaping a new scenario in the country, in which the incidence of chronic non-communicable diseases has been growing, including in the younger segments, becoming an increasing problem within quilombola communities (GUERRERO, 2010).

Traditional indigenous communities and quilombo remnants are currently considered to be groups of high social vulnerability, due to the historical issues suffered by their ancestors. In these groups, poverty, lack of sufficient income, scarcity of natural resources, hunger and food insecurity are highly prevalent and have major consequences for the state of health and life. However, this situation tends to improve with the creation of proper policies aimed at these traditional communities, the establishment of programs such as the National School Feeding Program aimed at these traditional communities, the establishment of programs such as the National School Feeding Program (CARVALHO, 2010).

The National School Feeding Program (PNAE), created in 1954, is the oldest and largest food and nutrition program in Brazil. Its aim is to meet the nutritional needs of students in basic education and youth and adult education, by providing food supplements while they are in the classroom, contributing to their growth, development, learning and school performance, as well as promoting the formation of healthy eating habits (SANTOS, et al 2008).

In traditional communities such as the quilombolas, there has been evidence of a serious situation of food insecurity which is associated with the constant threat to the control and preservation of their territories, where they carry out their subsistence activities, and the precarious access to public policies (BRASIL, 2005). It is estimated that around 129,000 quilombola children in the country are served by the PNAE and that, for many of them, school meals are their only daily meal. However, although these children may be protected against malnutrition, food insecurity threatens and affects their families (PEREIRA, 2009).

There are 35 quilombola communities in Sergipe, of which Mussuca in Laranjeiras and Patioba in Japaratuba are the largest. According to Laranjeiras (2006), the Mussuca settlement is characterized as follows: estimated population of 2,000 inhabitants; public transport linking the settlement to the capital; approximately 600 families living in the settlement; two schools, one municipal (the largest: where our research subjects are) and the other state (in the process of being municipalized); health post and soccer pitch; electricity network and most of the streets paved with cobblestones. There is piped water in the community. In terms of culture, Mussuca has elements that give it, as the Centro Laranjeirense de Cultura e Desenvolvimento - Celacude (Laranjeirense Center for Culture and Development) puts it, the identity of "a little piece of Africa" in Sergipe: Sao Gonzalo, Samba de Coco and Samba de Pareia are strong elements of popular culture in the village.

According to Silva et al, (2008), in their study of quilombola communities in Santarém, Pará, they identified that these communities recognize that they are in a situation of food insecurity and consider the most important causal factors for this to be the lack of land ownership. According to the conceptions of these communities, the fact that quilombola land is not titled can influence the nutritional status of the communities because of the way in which food is supplied, available, accessed and consumed.

In their study of quilombola communities in Bahia, Soares and Barreto (2014) indicate that overweight and abdominal obesity are important health problems in quilombola communities and, more specifically, among women. The prevalence of overweight and obesity was higher among quilombola women.

3.2. . Overweight and Obesity

The terms overweight and obesity are not synonymous and have different definitions which in many ways meet. The classification of overweight and obesity provides "meaningful comparisons of weight status within and between populations; the identification of individuals and groups at greatest risk of morbidity and mortality; the identification of priorities for intervention at community and individual levels and a firm basis for evaluating interventions" (WHO, 2004). Barros (2011) defined obesity as a chronic, progressive, fatal, genetically related disease characterized not only by the excessive accumulation of fat, but also by the development of other diseases (co-morbidities).

Obesity is characterized by the excessive accumulation of body fat with potential damage to health. According to the WHO (1998), various factors can interact in its etiology, such as genetic, environmental, dietary and physical activity patterns and individual biological factors, among many others. Obesity is not synonymous with being overweight, but rather with greater fat deposits (Domingues, 2000).

The most widely accepted definition of obesity is that which states that it is a quantity of total body fat, which represents one of the components of body weight, above normal standards (POLLOCK et al., 1986). According to the World Health Organization (WHO, 2004), obesity is a "disease in which excess body fat has accumulated to such an extent that health may be affected".

Obesity is classified as endogenous (primary), derived from hormonal problems, and exogenous (nutritional or secondary), resulting from an imbalance in the "metabolic balance" between calorie intake and expenditure, which should be treated with dietary guidance and adequate and targeted physical activity (MEYER; MELLO and LUFT, 2004). According to Fisberg (2005), exogenous obesity accounts for 95% of cases and endogenous obesity only 5%.

According to (MIRANDA, 2006) obesity is a chronic degenerative disease that currently affects both adults and children. It is interesting to identify it because its sufferers can present increased risks of morbidity and mortality, since it appears as one of the main causes of various chronic and non-infectious diseases, such as cardiovascular, gastrointestinal, hypertension and certain types of cancer.

Obesity, according to (APN, 2011; WHO, 2014), due to the excess of accumulated body fat, can reach proportions capable of affecting health. Excess fat is considered to be the result of successive positive energy balances, i.e. an amount of energy ingested through food consumption that is greater than the amount of energy expended (DGS, 2013). Excessive calorie intake and reduced physical activity also contribute significantly to this positive energy balance and consequently to the development of the disease, especially when they act together (RIBEIRO, 2008).

Obesity today has become synonymous with a sedentary lifestyle and a high-calorie diet, which can all be associated with a number of predisposing factors, including genetic factors, although these only account for a small percentage of responsibility (SOUSA, 2011; CDC, 2013).

Obesity has been linked to the appearance of respiratory problems, dermatological disorders, locomotor system disorders, dyslipidemia, increased tendency to blood clotting, insulin resistance, type 2 diabetes mielittus, sleep apnea, among others (Leao et al. 2003).

3.3. Childhood Obesity

Childhood has always been known as a time of great energy, when children play, run, jump and even tumble and fall. In the 21st century, however, we are seeing a new group of children: sedentary, less healthy, more prone to developing diseases, particularly obesity (TOEWS et al, 2004).

Among the various factors considered responsible for making a child obese, the following have been highlighted: consumption of inadequate food, lack of physical activity, anxiety, depression, hormonal and genetic factors, the change in behavior of modern society with the excessive use of computers and video games making them sedentary, as well as the low consumption of foods considered healthy, (MOURA et al, 2012).

Soares and Petroski (2003) reported that there are three periods in life when an increase in the number of fat cells (fat cell hyperplasia) can occur: the last trimester of pregnancy, when the mother's eating habits can change the body composition of the developing fetus; the first year of life; and the adolescent growth spurt (estirao).

Children's accelerated weight gain has been used to predict their later risk of developing obesity. However, it is not clear what factors influence the diet and weight gain of these children. It is known that energy intake during childhood determines weight gain and can influence the risk of developing obesity in adolescence and adulthood (GILMAR et al, 2010).

In their study carried out through a bibliographic survey of the Med Line and Lilacs systems (from 1995 to 2003), Luiz et al (2005) found that there is a possible relationship between childhood obesity and psychological aspects such as depression, anxiety and social competence deficits. For these authors, there are indications of correlations between these psychological aspects and the presence of obesity in children.

The mechanism of obesity is quite complex and there is not one factor, but a set of factors which, when combined, can lead to the onset of obesity at increasingly early ages (COUTO, 2015). These factors include genetic, metabolic, environmental and behavioral factors (BRASIL, 2005; REGO et al, 2007; MARTINS, 2008; NUNES, 2008; SOUSA, 2011; CDC, 2013).

The prevalence of obesity in children and adolescents has increased alarmingly worldwide. In 2013, it was estimated that there were around 43 million obese children under the age of 5, of which around 35 million lived in developed countries and the remaining 8 million in developing countries (ONIS et al, 2010; WHO, 2014). The scenario in Europe is not much more encouraging, as it is believed that there are around 14 million overweight children, 3 million of whom are obese (EASO, 2013; DUARTE, 2011; DGS, 2012). It is estimated that around twenty percent of school-age children in Europe will be overweight with an increased risk of developing chronic diseases when they become adults. Of these overweight children, one in five will be obese, with a significant probability that they are already suffering the first signs of cardiovascular disease, diabetes and liver disease (EASO, 2013).

According to data from EASO (2013), Portugal occupies a worrying position in Europe when it comes to the prevalence of overweight in children. Among Portuguese children aged 2 to 5, 26% are overweight and 12.5% are obese. Among children aged between 6 and 8, 32% are overweight and 13.9% are obese (EASO, 2013; APCOI, 2014). In Coimbra, (RITO, 2004), 2400 pre-school children aged between 3 and 6 were assessed and the following findings were described: 23.6% were overweight, of which 16.9% were pre-obese and 6.7% were obese. In this study, female children were the most pre-obese and obese. Another study on this subject

(MOREIRA, 2007) carried out a similar study, also in the Coimbra region, in which only male children aged between 2 and 6 were included in the sample, and found a prevalence of pre-obesity and obesity of 20.6% and 7.8%, respectively.

In the United States, there are major disparities in obesity between sociodemographic groups (WANG, 2011). According to (OGDEN, et al. 2014), childhood obesity is becoming a national (US) public health crisis. The author reported that in 2011-2012, the prevalence of obesity in the United States was 16.9% in young people and 34.9% in adults, respectively. OGDEN also reported that at 20112012, 31.8% (95% CI, 29.1%-34.7%) of young Americans were overweight or obese, and 16.9% (95% CI, 14.9%-19.2%) were obese.

According to Nagle et al (2013), data collected in Bolivia, Brazil, Colombia, Mexico, Paraguay and Peru put overweight rates for children at 12.2 to 23.9% and estimates of childhood obesity at 1.8 to 4.7%. According to the author, Latin American countries have some of the highest rates of overweight preschool children and, as a whole, Latin America has the highest proportion of overweight preschoolers compared to developing countries in Africa and Asia.

The results of national health surveys in 71 countries suggest that the proportion of overweight and obese preschoolers in Latin America is approaching the proportions found in the USA, as there are some Latin American countries with rates of more than 20% of overweight children between the ages of 5 and 17. In Brazil this rate is estimated at 21.1% for girls and 23.1% for boys; in Mexico 29% for girls and 28.1% for boys[7] and 27.1% for girls and 28.6% for boys in Chile. In Colombia, the rates increased from 10.3% to 17.5% between 2005 and 2010.

According to Eisenberg et al (2013), among developing countries, Mexico is becoming the most obese nation in the world. Its obesity rates are now the second highest in the world, followed by the United States. United States (USA). According to Shamah-Levy T; Villalpando-Hernández; Rivera-Dommarco; (2007), the Encuesta Nacional de Salud y Nutrición 2006 (ENSANUT; Mexican National Health and Nutrition Survey), the prevalence of overweight and obesity in Mexico for children aged 5 to 11 is around 26.0%, which represented an increase of 39.7% compared to 1999.

In Brazil, according to Gilmar et al (2010), in recent years, at the same time as there has been a drop in the occurrence of malnutrition in certain subgroups and regions of the country, the rise of overweight and obesity in the population has been highlighted as important public health problems. This establishes a coexistence of temporal trends between malnutrition and obesity, thus defining one of the defining characteristics of the country's nutritional transition process.

According to Abrantes et al. (2002), geographical differences also express differences in the genesis of overweight and obesity. They point to a higher prevalence of overweight and obesity in higher income regions, which explains the differences in the epidemiological panorama between the Northeast and Southeast of Brazil.

However, it is worth noting that, in recent years, another trend has already emerged: an increase in the occurrence of obesity in low-income regions (BATISTA and RISSIN, 2003).

In Brazil, the number of people who are overweight or obese has grown, according to the Vigitel survey (BRASIL, 2014), which indicated that 52.5% of Brazilians are overweight, which was 43% in 2006, and 17.9% of the population is obese. This same survey showed that there has been a 23% increase in the last nine years.

With regard to the prevention and treatment of obesity, it is essential to use a reliable method that can reliably identify its presence. In this context, the use of the Body Mass Index (BMI) has been strongly accepted by the scientific community involved in the study of obesity, due to its easy application and statistical relationship with total body fat in young people (KOCHI, 2004 TADDEI, 2000).

A study carried out by researchers from the Departments of Nutrition at the Federal University of Pernambuco (UFPE) and Alagoas (UFA) investigated the prevalence of overweight and its association with socioeconomic, biological and maternal factors in children under five years of age in the semi-arid region of the state of Alagoas, which is characterized by poor public service infrastructure and poor social indicators (MOREIRA et al., 2012). A total of 963 children under the age of 5 were assessed, with a homogeneous distribution in relation to gender. Of these, 51.4% were male and the average age was 27.7 months (standard deviation ± 17.3). The study shows that 192 children (19.9%) are at risk of being overweight, 63 (6.5%) are overweight and 20 (2.1%) are obese.

According to Ezzati (2016), "The number of people in the world whose weight poses a serious threat to health has never been higher". The study revealed an alarming increase in obesity rates over the last 40 years, finding that the number of people with a BMI over 30 has risen from 105 million in 1975 to 641 million in 2014. More than one in ten men and one in seven women are obese.

1.4 - Body Mass Index

According to the WHO (2004) BMI can be considered the most useful measure for providing data on obesity at a population level. Although it is a measure that does not distinguish between fat and muscle weight, it can be used to estimate the prevalence of obesity in a population and the risks associated with it, because the small number of people who are overweight due to their large muscle mass are disregarded when the number of people assessed is large. The percentage of fat derived from skinfolds is impractical epidemiologically (COLE et al., 2000) and body mass and height are simple measures with high reproducibility and a high but not total correlation with the amount of body fat (GUEDES et al., 2006). The use of BMI to identify overweight and obese adults is consensual (GUEDES et al., 2006; WHO, 2004; ABRANTES et al., 2002), and its cut-off points (25 kg/m2 for overweight and 30 kg/m2 for obesity) allow comparisons between and within populations (GUEDES et al., 2006).

However, its use in the nutritional assessment of children and adolescents does not occur in the same way. BMI became more widespread after Must et al. (1991) published percentile values for age and sex (ABRANTES et al., 2003). The difficulties related to the lack of consensus on the cut-off points to be used stem from the fact that height is still increasing at this stage, and body composition is continually in transition, as well as differences between ethnic groups (WHO, 2004).

BMI has therefore been used in national and international studies and has been chosen as the method for designating the prevalence of overweight and obese children, along with the cut-off points proposed by Cole et al (2000).

1.5 - Health problems related to obesity

Obesity in children has numerous health complications (DGS, 2005; ONIS, et al, 2010; RÊGO, 2010). The consequences imposed by this disease affect the human organism at the level of all the systems of the human body (SOARES; PETROSKI, 2003; RÊGO, 2010). These complications inherent to the disease lie in the persistence of risky behavior into adulthood (OPPERMAN; CASSANDRA, 2001).

Psychological disorders are one of the most visible consequences in obese children. These children have a lack of self-esteem, problems with social integration, isolation, suffer from *bullying,* and this can be reflected in situations such as depression (OPPERMAN; CASSANDRA, 2001; SOARES; PETROSKI, 2003; COELHO; BRAGANÇA, 2005).

Obesity generates dissatisfaction with body image and non-acceptance of the body, which can lead people to feel excluded from society. In this way, children and adolescents who are faced with obesity have many problems in terms of acceptance, self-esteem and valuing their own bodies (FERRIANI et al, 2005).

With regard to psychosocial factors, the disparagement of one's own physical image is a very frequent finding, which generates insecurity in relation to the social group. Overweight and obese children often refer to their weight as an aggravating factor in social interaction, suffering discrimination that interferes with their social and emotional relationships (GIULIANO and CARNEIRO, 2004).

According to Luiz et al (2005), when they analyzed the scientific literature, they found a relationship between childhood obesity and psychological aspects such as depression, anxiety and deficits in social competence. For these authors, there are indications of correlations between these psychological aspects and the presence of obesity in children.

Childhood obesity is the main cardiovascular risk factor in adulthood, and is associated with a sedentary lifestyle and incorrect eating habits, favoring various diseases and increasing mortality. Another relevant risk factor is arterial hypertension, which is on the rise among children and can be secondary to other diseases or even primary or essential, of idiopathic cause, being associated with obesity (REZENDE, 2014).

According to Feldmann et al (2012), children need to feel loved, respected and valued. Generally, the lack of these aspects occurs within the family itself, and not just at school or in the social environment in which they live. If a child grows up with good physical, psychological and social support, they will cope better with life's adversities and will have many more internal resources to do so.

1.6 - Nutrition and environmental factors related to obesity

According to (DE CARVALHO, 2014), the health standards of a population will be low whenever nutrition is inadequate. Therefore, nutrition and food education are fundamental determinants, along with health care, preventive medicine and public health.

Environmental factors are increasingly being linked to childhood weight gain and overweight in genetically stable populations, as associated socioeconomic and demographic conditions modify the family environment where some children tend to develop overweight more easily than others (MULDER et al., 2009). These factors include, among others, the availability and accessibility of healthy foods, dietary practices or sedentary behavior, family meals, television use during meals, eating out and portion size, time and financial constraints, traditional and cultural methods of food preparation, parental food preferences, nutritional knowledge and the child's eating practices (CULLEN et al., 2001; GOLAN; CROW; 2004; PATRICK; NICKLAS, 2005; VETRINI, 2009).

Over time, eating habits have been changing and the environment in which children and adolescents are inserted favors inappropriate eating behaviors, such as caloric snacks, increased frequency of meals and low consumption of fruit and vegetables and high in calories, refined carbohydrates and saturated fat consumed by parents (JIANG et al., 2005; MORENO; RODRIGUEZ, 2007; MOTA et al., 2008).

Adequate food and nutrition are essential requirements for children's growth and development. They are fundamental human rights, as they represent the basis of life itself. In order to be well nourished, children and adolescents need a variety of safe foods in sufficient quantity and of good quality (MINISTÉRIO DA SAÚDE, 2000).

The main aim of food education is to encourage and establish healthy eating practices. Through food education in schools, it is possible to introduce desirable eating attitudes at a stage when habits and personality traits are not yet very solid. Parental cooperation is essential in this regard. Children and adolescents need simple, objective and direct information about food that helps them understand their nutritional needs (BURTON, 1979).

According to Sawaya and Filgueiras (2013), a people's diet has always been one of the most specific characteristics of each culture since the beginning. Despite this, the food industry and trade have developed techniques for selling and inducing new eating habits that have been able to overcome the profound cultural influence of each people when eating. More recently, they have been able to develop flavors, images and persuasion techniques to reach children from all social classes and change their habits and those of their families.

Foods rich in sugar, fat and salt generate positive emotions more than other foods, which increase the motivation to obtain them as soon as they are remembered or are available at hand, in other words, eating them is *rewarding*. Our bodies have developed a particular appetite for them, as they guarantee greater availability of energy like sugar and fat, while salt guarantees the hydroelectrolytic balance that is vital for the body to function (SAWAYA and FILGUEIRAS 2013).

Foods rich in these ingredients can maintain their stimulating effect over a longer period of time through the more prolonged release of *dopamine* by the hedonic system. Animal studies have shown that the release of this neurotransmitter does not undergo the habituation process when highly palatable foods are ingested compared to less palatable ones such as normal food (NORGREN et al., 2006).

This phenomenon shows that the body sees advantages in eating these foods over others, and inhibits the process of habituation, favoring consumption whenever the opportunity arises. Dopamine release is greater if the palatable food is offered in small quantities intermittently, if the animal can anticipate its offer by some recognizable environmental signal, or if the schedule is maintained each day. The degree of palatability of a food is calculated by the intensity of the hedonic perception of the oral sensory signals (aroma, taste, image, texture) caused by it (YEOMANS,1998).

Children become obese due to various factors, including the consumption of inadequate food, lack of physical activity, anxiety, depression, hormonal and genetic factors, the change in behavior of modern society with the excessive use of computers and video games making them sedentary, as well as the low consumption of foods considered healthy, (MOURA et al. 2012).

Other factors are also associated with low-quality food consumption in children. In the city of Vitória - Espirito Santo, a cross-sectional study was carried out with 1282 school-age children and found that poor diet quality was associated with low maternal schooling (OR=3.93; 95% CI: 2.58;5.99), absence of the father in the household (OR=2.03; 95% CI: 1.68;2.99) and not having lunch at the table (OR=1.47; 95% CI: 1.12;1.93), (MOLINA et al., 2010).

The role of the television media, with its bombardment of advertisements for food products, has also been reported as influencing maternal choices. Borzekowski et al, (2001), reported that eating patterns are changing and that these changes are closely related to the habit of watching television. According to these authors, just 30 seconds' exposure to food commercials can influence food choices, leading to greater consumption of foods rich in fats and sugars which, in general, are the ones most often shown on this media. Bener et al. found a strong association between children who spent hours on the computer or watching TV and eating fast food, leading to the development of inadequate eating habits (BENER et al., 2010). In Manchester, England, Shi and Mao (2010) found that an increase in the frequency of consumption of fast food and sugary drinks was present in adolescents who spent > 2 hours a day watching television (SHI; MAO, 2010).

Fiates; Amboni and Teixeira in 2008, in the city of Florianópolis, investigated the relationship between children's food choices and their relationship with watching television and physical activity. They found that the more children watched television, the higher their consumption of high-calorie foods.

Children are considered to be the most vulnerable group to unhealthy food advertising, as they are less informed and less able to judge the messages being broadcast (HENRIQUES et al., 2012). However, when television is used as an educational vehicle, children are also the ones who respond best, as shown in a study in Houston, Texas, when Nicklas and Cols, in 2010, checked whether fruit and vegetable commercials have a positive impact on children's preferences and the result met expectations, proving that there was a positive influence on children's food preferences for fruit and vegetables (NICKLAS et al., 2010).

Thus, (AQUINO; PHILIPPI; 2002; MOLINA et al., 2010), emphasized that in order to promote lasting changes in children's diets and, consequently, possible improvements in health, it must be understood that the family represents the first and most important link in promoting healthy eating and that the parents' decision determines not only the child's food intake, but also the food choices that will influence the formation of eating habits.

1.7 - Physical activity

Lifestyle is closely associated with health and quality of life for people of all ages. The habits and choices that define an individual's lifestyle are largely established before adulthood and it is believed that the factors that contribute to the acquisition of certain behaviors stem from the physical and social environment in which one lives (NAHAS et al., 2003). According to Alves (2003), the acquisition of knowledge and positive attitudes such as physical activity, proper nutrition and preventive behaviors are consolidated during childhood and youth.

Although physical activity is of fundamental importance in children's lives, there has been an increasing tendency to adopt hypokinetic behavioural patterns, characterized by a predominance of passive leisure activities (watching television and electronic games) to the detriment of more vigorous physical activities (HALLAL et al., 2010; TENÓRIO et al., 2010).

The lack of physical activity and excessive exposure to sedentary behavior observed in preschool children has been associated with negative health outcomes such as being overweight and, later on, with cardiovascular diseases (JANZ et al., 2009). Meanwhile, the regular practice of physical activity can prevent the onset of obesity, as well as benefiting the prevention and treatment of diabetes, metabolic syndrome and lipid profile, and also benefiting the health-related quality of life of obese children and adolescents (CHEN; ROBERTS; BARNARD, 2006; FULLERTON et al., 2007; SATO et al., 2007; LEITE et al, 2009).

Monzavi et al. found positive effects of physical exercise, through recreational activities, and nutritional guidance on the components of metabolic syndrome (MONZAVI et al., 2006) and Alves et al. on the body mass index of obese children (ALVES et al., 2008).

Poeta and Cols, (2013) aimed to examine the effects of an intervention program with recreational activities and nutritional guidance on the health-related quality of life of obese children. The authors found that the interdisciplinary intervention was effective in reducing BMI and improving quality of life in the physical, emotional, social, psychosocial and general quality of life domains. They also showed the multiple benefits of an intervention program with recreational activities and nutritional guidance, in addition to conventional treatment for obese children. The quality of life indicator was also highly relevant during the planning of actions to control childhood obesity, due to its role in assessing the effects of treatment and maintaining healthy habits, thus favoring treatment adherence, obesity control and the prevention of recurrence in the medium and long term.

Chapter 4

4. - METHODOLOGY

4.1 Study design

This is a cross-sectional study with an exploratory and quantitative approach.

4.2 Place of study

Laranjeiras is a Brazilian municipality in the state of Sergipe. It is located at latitude 10°48'23" south and longitude 37°10'12" west, at an altitude of 9 meters. According to IBGE data (2012), the population of the municipality in 2010 was estimated at 26,902 inhabitants. It has an area of 163.4 km^2 . The Mussuca quilombola community is located in the municipality of Laranjeiras, situated in Baixo Cotinguiba, a micro-region in the east of the state of Sergipe. It is easily accessible via the BR 101, Sergipe's main highway, and is 19 km from Aracaju, the state capital. It has ups and downs, with a relief of tableland, with differences and composition of hills embedded in slopes.

According to data from the municipal health department, the quilombola population of Mussuca is approximately 3,043. The majority of this population defines itself as black, which has always been linked to the presence of slave labor and currently to sugarcane cultivation. The local economy is based on fishing, agriculture, mineral extraction and the public sector, in the case of the town hall, more specifically the big companies, where there are far more jobs on offer. The lack of sustainability in the community means that most of these individuals move to the capital and neighboring towns and even to other states.

Mussuca has two public schools, one state and the other municipal, a telephone and electricity network, a health center, a cemetery, a sports court, a gym, untreated drinking water, paved streets, a soccer field, evangelical and Catholic churches, community and fishermen's associations, among others. A digital telecenter, Umbanda centers, a daycare center that doesn't work and local businesses.

The Prefeito José Monteiro Sobral Municipal School in the village of Mussuca, founded on February 9, 1988, through Municipal Law No. 083, sanctioned by the Laranjeiras City Council, is part of the Laranjeiras municipal education network. The school offers Early Childhood Education, Primary Education and Youth and Adult Education. The school is well located and easily accessible. It caters for a target audience of 440 pupils, 85% of whom are students from the quilombola community of Mussuca and 15% from 10 surrounding villages. The school caters for kindergarten, primary and secondary education.

The school's primary and secondary schools are divided into morning, afternoon and evening shifts. They were selected for this study because they represent children and adolescents from one of the largest quilombola communities in Sergipe.

4.3 Sample selection.

The BMI data was collected from all the students aged between 5 and 14 at the municipal school in the community and the information from the questionnaire was collected in the field from the students' parents or guardians.

According to the school census (INEP, 2014), the number of students enrolled in elementary school in the 5-14 age group was 301.

The calendar year was used, where the lower age is the year of birth and the upper age is the year of the survey. All students between the ages of 5 and 14 who were regularly enrolled at the school were pre-selected. However, participation in the study was conditional on the following: authorization from parents or guardians to take part in the study and the students agreeing to take part. The exclusion criterion was the presence of any physical or mental disability.

4.4 Study variables

- Dependent variables: Childhood Obesity, BMI Index;

To analyze the presence of overweight and obesity, using the height and weight of each child, BMI was calculated, which according to the Ministry of Health protocol (2006) is grouped into four classes: BMI percentile greater than 95 indicates obesity; BMI percentile between 85 and 95 means pre-obesity; BMI percentile greater than 5 and less than 85 represents a normal state and BMI percentile less than 5 means thinness.

- Independent variables: sociodemographic, economic;

Miranda's (2006) questionnaire was used to assess the following parameters: gender, age, weaning age, reference by parents or guardians of obesity in the child, identification of the family as obese, whether the child has a habit of drinking water, regularity of meal times, intake of liquids during meals, number of meals/day, dessert habit, frequency of soft drink intake, fast food, family tries to re-educate, use of food rewards for good behavior, parents work outside, caregiver for children in the absence of parents, bullying by family, bullying by friends, recent trauma, leisure time at weekends, television, video games or computer time and physical activity outside school.

4.5 Instruments and procedures

A *Filizola* electronic scale was used to obtain the weight measurements. The children were weighed using a single measurement in an orthostatic position, standing on the scale, barefoot and wearing school clothes, a procedure adopted by some authors in similar studies (LEÂO et al, 2003; DE SOUZA, 2003). To measure the children's height, a vertical stadiometer was used and their height was recorded in centimeters.

4.6 Ethical aspects

From an ethical point of view, the project complied with CNS Resolution 466/12 and was approved by the Ethics Committee (CEP/UNIT) under process no. 1.722.083 (Appendix 1).

4.7 Self-administered questionnaire

The questionnaire drawn up by Miranda (2006), which was validated by the Ethics Committee for Research with Human Beings at the Adventist University of São Paulo, was used because of the need to find out about the children's lives outside of school, as it was necessary to delineate more specifically what the students' lifestyle habits were, together with those of their families, in order to compare them with the data obtained from the physical assessment. For ethical reasons, the identity of the participants was preserved. The questionnaire drawn up by Miranda (2006) was used and validated. It was considered that this instrument could also be used for the quilombola community of Mussuca, which, due to its proximity to the city of Laranjeiras and the state capital, may or may not have similar characteristics to non-quilombola communities.

4.8 Statistical Analysis

The information collected was described using simple frequencies and percentages. Associations were tested using Pearson's chi-square test. The significance level adopted was 5% and the software used was R Core Team 2016.

RESULTS

The results of this study are presented in the form of two original articles.

Article 1 submitted in accordance with Annex II

Overweight and obesity prevalence among children and adolescents in the Quilombo Community of Mussuca of Laranjeiras - Sergipe

Luciano S. Teixeira[1] ; Erasmo A. Junior[2] ; Francisco P. Reis[3]

[1]Student Department of the Master Course Department of Graduate Health and Environment, University Tiradentes, Av Murilo Dantas, 300 49032-490 - Farolandia, Aracaju - SE, Brazil; E-mail: lucianoteixeira_2@hotmail.com;
[2]Doctor UFBA, Rua Alferes Pedro de Brito, 100, 49032-010 - Farolandia, Aracaju - SE, Brazil; E-mail: anatjjunior@ig.com.br
[3]Professor the Department of Medicine at the University Tiradentes (Supervisor). Rua Silvio César Leite, 301,49020-060 - Salgado Filho, Aracaju - SE, Brazil; E-mail:franciscopradoreis@gmail.com

Correspondence to: Luciano

Sousa Teixeira E-mail: lucianoteixeira_2@hotmail.com

Introduction

Quilombocommunitiesare
remaining populations of old quilombos, and is a representation of the resistance of black Brazilians. They are a lot of located in various regions of the country, especially in rural areas there was a relative degree of geographical isolation and live significant social usually population health inequalities (Monego 2010).

These communities bear a great historical complexity to be the result of resistance to the process of slavery imposed for centuries on blacks and that even after the Golden Law remain marginalized by society (Salles 2005).

Many quilombos, after the abolition of slavery led to the current Quilombo communities. The members of these

communities have strong cultural ties, maintaining their traditions

, religious practices, relationship with work on earth and system of social organization (Carvalho, 1995).

From a legal point of view, quilombo communities were officially recognized by the Brazilian State in 1988, Article # 68 of the Transitory Constitutional Provisions Act (Brazil 2002).

The traditional indigenous and quilombo communities are currently considered highly vulnerable social groups, for historical issues suffered by their ancestors. In these groups, poverty, lack of sufficient income, scarcity of natural resources, hunger and food insecurity, are highly prevalent and with great consequences for health and life. However, this situation tends to improve with the creation of policies themselves directed at these traditional communities, institution programs such as the National School Feeding Programme (Carvalho, 2010).

Specifically from the health point of view, we can see the process of nutritional and epidemiological transition shaping a new scenario in the country, where the incidence of chronic communicable diseases is growing, even in the younger segments and it is going to be a problem rising within the quilombola communities (Guerrero, 2010).

Childhood obesity is a current problem with several implications for human life. An obese child is more likely to come to develop diseases later in life, which hinder you both personal and social life. According to Spence; Lee (2003) during the last two decades, changes in the social and economic structure of society and the processes of modernization, urbanization and all the technological innovations brought about changes in daily habits.

Obesity is a disease that the accumulated excess body fat can reach proportions that could affect health (APN 2011; WHO, 2014). Excessive fat results from successive positive energy balance, i.e. the amount of energy consumed by food consumption is greater than the amount of energy expended (DGS, 2013). Excessive intake of high-calorie foods, and reduced physical activity contribute significantly to this positive energy balance and consequently to the development of this disease, especially when they act together (Ribeiro, 2008).

Actually obesity is synonymous of inactivity and a high calorie diet, however, it was well associated with this set of predisposing factors for its development and also genetic factors may be included, although these represent a small percentage of responsibility (Sousa, 2011; CDC, 2013).

Childhood has always been known as a great power stage, where children play, run, jump, fall, however, in the XXI century we are seeing a new group of children: sedentary children, less healthy children, more children prone to developing diseases, including the development of obesity (Tows et al, 2004).

Children become obese due to several factors, among which stands out the consumption of unsuitable foods, lack of physical activity anxiety, depression, hormonal and genetic factors, a change in behavior of modern society with excessive use of computers and video games making them sedentary, in addition to low consumption of foods considered healthy, (Moura et al. 2012).

The prevalence rates of obesity have increased alarmingly and span the globe. In 2013, it was estimated that there were about 43 million obese children under 5 years, and about 35 million lived in developed countries and the remaining 8 million in developing countries (ONIS et al, 2010; WHO, 2014). The scenario in Europe is not much more encouraging, as it is believed that there are approximately 14 million overweight children, and 3 million are obese (EASO, 2013; Duarte, 2011; DGS, 2012). Twenty percent of school-age children in Europe are estimated to be overweight with an increased risk of developing chronic diseases as they become adults. Of these children are overweight, one in five are obese, with a significant probability that they are already experiencing early signs of cardiovascular disease, diabetes and liver disease (EASO, 2013).

In the United States there are large disparities in obesity among sociodemographic groups (Wang, 2011). Childhood obesity has become a national public health crisis, because in 20112012, the prevalence of obesity in the United States was 16.9% of young people and 34.9% in adults, although the prevalence remained stable between 2003-2004 and 2009-2010 (OGDEN, 2012). In 2011-2012, 31.8% (95% CI, 29.1% -34.7%) of young people were overweight or obese, and 16.9% (95% CI, 14.9% -19.2%) of the youth were obese. In 2011-2012, there was no difference in the prevalence of obesity among boys and girls (OGDEN, 2012).

Second (Nagle, 2013), data collected in Bolivia, Brazil, Colombia, Mexico, Paraguay and Peru put the rates of overweight children from 12.2 to 23.9% and childhood obesity estimates from 1.8 to 4.7% . Latin American countries have some of the highest rates of preschool children with overweight and, as a whole, Latin America had the highest proportion of preschool overweight children, compared to the developing countries in Africa and Asia. The results of national health surveys from 71 countries suggest that the proportion of preschool children with overweight and obesity in Latin America is approaching proportions found in the US with more than 20% of overweight children in some Latin American countries rates obesity for children 5-17 years in Brazil are 21.1% for girls and 23.1 % for boys, 29% for girls and 28.1% for boys in Mexico, and 27.1% of girls and 28.6 % for boys in Chile are obese ones. In Colombia, the rates increased from children 10.3% to 17.5% between 2005 and 2010.

According to the study (Eisenerg 2013), developing countries, like Mexico, are becoming one of the most obese in the world. Obesity rates in Mexico are now the second largest in the world, following the United States (US). According to the Encuesta Nacional de Salud y Nutrición 2006 (ENSANUT, National Mexican Health and Nutrition Survey), the prevalence of overweight and obesity in Mexico for children 5-11 is about 26.0%, which is an increase of 39.7% over 1999.

In Brazil, according to (Gilmar et al. 2010), in recent years, while there was a decrease in the occurrence of malnutrition in certain subgroups and Country Regions, the ascendancy of overweight and obesity in the population has been increasing as important public health problems. It is established, thus coexistence of temporal trends between malnutrition and obesity, thereby defining one of the striking features of the nutritional transition process of the country.

Thus, the present study was to evaluate the prevalence of Obesity in Children and Youth groups of children from five to fourteen years of a Quilombo Community in public network School Laranjeiras-SE, Brazil.

Materials and Methods

This is a cross-sectional study with a quantitative approach developed during the second half of 2016 in a quilombola community in the municipality of Laranjeiras - SE to Mussuca. The study population consisted of 301 students aged between 5 and 14 years living in Mussuca community. In this community live on average 600 families and the main source of income is fishing and industries in neighboring towns.

The study included children and adolescents who agreed 5 to 14 years old to participate by signing the

Consent Term, in addition to the Consent and Informed signed by parents or guardians. The exclusion criteria, subjects who had a got any diseases that prevent cold the student from participating in the study.

The collection of anthropometric data was performed at the select school where they also study by apytying aplying questionnaires taken home for the responsible answer. Contact the community was conducted by Director of the municipal school.

The questionnaire was used (Miranda 2006), to evaluate the sociodemographic and nutritional status of respondents, there was measurement of weight and height for the subsequent calculation of body mass index (BMI).

Data were described by simple and percentage frequencies. Association was tested using the Pearson chi-square test. The significance level was 5% and the software used was R Core Team 2016. This study complied with the ethical precepts, was approved by the Research Ethics Committee of the University Tiradentes, under the number 1722083, obeying all the commandments of Resolution 466/2012 (14) of the National Health Council at all stages of its implementation.

Results

Figure 1 - School attendance by sex in the age group 5-14 years (N 301), Mussuca - SE 2016.

	Frequency	Valid percent
ValidMale	149	49,5
Female	152	50,5
Total	301	100,0

Figure 1 is showing the number of volunteers, girls and boys separately in the study. A total of 301 149 (49.5%) were male and 152 (50.5%) female.

Figure 2 - Frequency distribution of normal weight, overweight and obesity in the age group 5-14 years

school students (N 301), Mussuca - SE 2016.

	Age										X^2 (p-value)
	5	6	7	8	9	10	11	12	13	14	
Male											
BMI											
Eutrophic	5 (63)	3 (50)	5 (42)	12 (60)	9 (75)	9 (69)	15 (71)	12 (55)	13 (62)	8 (73)	17 (0,520)
Overweight	2 (25)	0 (0)	4 (33)	6 (30)	1 (8)	2 (15)	2 (10)	7 (32)	2 (10)	2 (18)	
Obesity	1 (13)	3 (50)	3 (25)	2 (10)	2 (17)	2 (15)	4 (19)	3 (14)	6 (29)	1 (9)	
Female											
BMI											
Eutrophic	3 (60)	3 (50)	6 (75)	6 (46)	13 (68)	8 (62)	14 (70)	12 (43)	22 (85)	10 (83)	26 (0,102)
Overweight	2 (40)	3 (50)	2 (25)	6 (46)	5 (26)	5 (38)	3 (15)	10 (36)	2 (8)	2 (17)	
Obesity	0 (0)	0 (0)	0 (0)	1 (8)	1 (5)	0 (0)	3 (15)	6 (21)	2 (8)	0 (0)	

Chi-square test

Figure 3 -
Distribution between BMI and daily habits of children and adolescents (N 301), Mussuca - SE 2016.

	BMI			
	eutrophic	overweight	obesity	X2 (p-value)
How many times a week does your child take soda?				
Once	64 (34)	8 (11,8)	5 (12,5)	71,2 (<0,001)
2 teams	41 (21,8)	6 (8,8)	2 (5)	
3 teams	73 (38,8)	36 (52,9)	13 (32,5)	
Others	10 (5,3)	18 (26,5)	20 (50)	
How many times a week does your child (a) eat out (Fast Food's)?				
Once	113 (60,1)	38 (55,9)	14 (35)	10,8 (0,093)
2 teams	34 (18,1)	9 (13,2)	10 (25)	
3 teams	26 (13,8)	13 (19,1)	9 (22,5)	
Others	15 (8)	8 (11,8)	7 (17,5)	
How much time per day, does it (a) watch television, play video games, or is in the computer?				
1 to 2 hours	46 (24,5)	15 (22,1)	3 (7,5)	37,4 (<0,001)
3 to 4 hours	103 (54,8)	21 (30,9)	13 (32,5)	
5 to 6 hours	26 (13,8)	24 (35,3)	14 (35)	
More than 7 hours	13 (6,9)	8 (11,8)	10 (25)	
Does your child do any physical activity, accompanied, extra school?				
Yes	84 (44,7)	7 (10,3)	5 (12,5)	35,3 (<0,001)

		BMI		
	eutrophic	overweight	obesity	X2 (p-value)
In	104 (55,3)	61 (89,7)	35 (87,5)	
If so, what?				
Swimming	4 (4,8)	0 (0)	2 (40)	14 (0,175)
Olympic gymnastics	2 (2,4)	0 (0)	0 (0)	
Dance	11 (13,1)	1 (14,3)	1 (20)	
Outhers	24 (28,6)	2 (28,6)	0 (0)	
Soccer	35 (41,7)	4 (57,1)	1 (20)	
Handball	8 (9,5)	0 (0)	1 (20)	

Figure 2 shows the number of volunteers, girls and boys assessing their nutritional status, eutrophic, overweight and obesity, aged 5-14 years. Observing the table above it can be seen that 62.5% of the volunteers are at normal weight and

35.9% already with changes in their anthropometric measurements. Of these, 108 (34.6%) are overweight, 40 (12.8%) already obese, as shown in the table,($p>0.05$)

Figure 3 shows the distribution between some habits of children and adolescents among them pointy to of soft drinks consumed weekly, snacking type (fast food's), average time in which participants are watching television or playing video games. It was observed that the participants overweight (79.4%) of refrigerants take three or more times a week, while participants taking obese refrigerant between three or more times a week is (80.5%). These high values in the intake of unhealthy foods are also evident when we analyze the item Snacking (fast food's) where (30.9%) of children and adolescents who are overweight consume this type of food among three or more times a week, while that among obese that number is even higher (39.5%) eat these types of food.

Still in Figure 3 shows the relationship between overweight and obesity and the time in which participants stand in front of the television, video game or computer. Among participants with overweight (47.1%) are more than five hours with this kind of entertainment, while the relationship with the obese it is much higher (60%) of respondents are more than five hours in front of these instruments. This may explain why these children and adolescents do not practice physical activities outside of school. Among the participants, with normal weight BMI (44.7%) responded that makes some kind of regular physical activity out of school, while the BMI overweight, only (10.3%) were told that some activity, and BMI obese (12.5%) reported participating in some physical activity.

Pearson Chi-square test

Discussion

In this study we analyzed the school as a whole, making no distinction between morning and daytime for analysis of obesity.

This study, with 301 volunteers to suggest that 108 (35.9%) of students are overweight, and of these 40 (13.3%) already obese.

It was found that obesity is prevalent in males and of thier age, the prevalence was 12 years for both sexes. At this age, 22 (15.1%) male volunteers participated in the survey, where 7 (25%) were overweight and 3 (11.1%) were already above 95 in the growth curve graph, so already degree of obesity.

The overweight rate and obesity together reaches 35.9% of the participants, making it clear that obesity is increasing every day.

In his work (Ferreira, 2011) evaluated 973 children (50.4% boys). Most families (60.8%) belonged to the class E (the poorest) and was assisted by the Bolsa Familia Program (76.0%). Householders had schooling < 4 years of education (75.9%) and 57.1% of households had more than 5 residents. The prevalence of PI deficits, PE, EI (decade ficit height) and overweight were respectively 3.4, 2.0, 11.5 and 7.1%. Anemia was identified in 52.7% of children and did not differ between those with stunting or overweight (P = 0.43).

Formerly fat was associated with health, but the number of malnourished children was greater than the obese, compared to today. We must remember that fear of violence was not so great and the food was much healthier. Industrialized products hardly exist and the children created their own play, which mostly were carried out on the street. The use of games and internet was not even an addiction among children and adolescents (Souza et al.).

In his work in a quilombo community in Santarem - PA, (Uchoa, 2014) concluded that the individuals surveyed by the body mass index (BMI), it was found that only 23.74% of the individuals are with ideal weight, while 19 % were overweight. Obesity It is characterized by almost 60% of the Maroons, the majority (28.6%) Class A, 23.9% are obese class two and class three 4.76% obese.

Lima et al (2004) concluded in his research with children and adolescents who were overweight and obese, poor diet with nutrient imbalance.

Mello et al, (2004), pointed out that when the child is forced to eat all that is offered, it may alter the development of their point of satiety, thereby increasing the risk for obesity.

The study showed as Figure 3, that 31.6% of children and adolescents have been more than 5 hours per day watching television or playing video games, thus confirming the number of children and adolescents who do not do any physical activity outside of school, 66.8% even as table 3.

Considering participation in physical activity, it can be said that only 66.8% of participants leads to a sedentary life, and the only activity is watching television and playing video games. Those who practice physical activity, mostly play football.

Mello et al (2004), in his research report that obese children tend to become sedentary, and that the activity carried out in the gym, is unlikely to be tolerated for a long time.

To spend energy are not required large investments but it is important to perform physical exercises. Habits such as up and down stairs, jumping rope, walking to school, playing hopscotch, are a great aid in the obesity fight, as

as well as a balanced diet. Recalling that diet and physical activity should be carried out simultaneously for the prevention and treatment of obesity.

Conclusions

This study, with 301 volunteers to suggest that 108 (35.9%) of students are overweight, and of these 40 (13.3%) already obese.

It was found that obesity is prevalent in males and of thier age, the prevalence was 12 years for both sexes.

At this age, 22 (15.1%) male volunteers participated in the survey, where 7 (25%) were overweight and 3 (11.1%) were already above 95 in the growth curve graph, so already degree of obesity. In women 28 (18.7%) 12 years old students who participated in the study and 10 (25%) students are overweight and 6 (46.2%) obese. Therefore, it is concluded that the most aggravating age for both sexes is, at age 12, where excess weight and obesity occurs.

Thanks - CAPES, FAPITEC - (PROMOB).

Article 2

EPIDEMIOLOGICAL PROFILE OF CHILDHOOD OBESITY IN A QUILOMBOLA COMMUNITY: RELATIONSHIP BETWEEN DAILY ELECTRONIC HABITS AND PHYSICAL ACTIVITY

Summary

It seems that the choice of a more sedentary lifestyle may be contributing to the increase in obesity among children and adolescents. Therefore, the main objective of this study was to investigate the epidemiological profile of obesity and overweight in school children and adolescents aged between 5 and 14, students from the 1st to the 9th grades at the Prefeito José Monteiro Municipal School, in the morning and afternoon shifts, located in the quilombola community of Mussuca - Laranjeiras - SE, and possible associations with daily habits of using electronic devices and practicing physical activity. The sample consisted of 301 children and adolescents of both sexes from this school group. Anthropometric measurements were taken of the children and questionnaires were administered to their parents. Analysis of the data collected allowed us to study the relationship between eating habits, physical activity and a sedentary lifestyle and the childhood obesity observed in the sample. 62.5% of the volunteers were considered normal weight and 35.9% already had changes in their anthropometric measurements. Of these, 108 (34.6%) are overweight, with 40 (12.8%) already obese, the number of volunteers, girls and boys assessing their nutritional status, eutrophic, overweight and obese, in the 5 to 14 age group.

KEYWORDS: childhood obesity; sedentary lifestyles; physical activity and television.

I - Introduction

Obesity is a disease in which excess accumulated body fat can reach proportions that can affect health (APN, 2011; WHO, 2014). Excess fat results from successive positive energy balances, i.e. the amount of energy ingested through food consumption is greater than the amount of energy expended (DGS, 2013). Excessive intake of caloric foods and reduced physical activity contribute significantly to this positive energy balance and consequently to the development of the disease, especially when they act together (RIBEIRO, 2008).

According to the World Health Organization (WHO) (1998) childhood obesity is defined as "A disease in which excess body fat has accumulated to such an extent that health may be affected". The WHO (2014) has classified obesity as "the epidemic of the century," in which there are millions of overweight people, hundreds of millions of obese people in the world, an increasing number of children and adolescents with obesity, a list of diseases associated with obesity that not only affects an increasing number, but also reaches more and more new people, spreading the epidemic not only in the most developed countries, but also in countries where just a few years ago hunger was not eradicated, and in vulnerable communities such as quilombolas.

Obesity, in its current state, has become synonymous with a sedentary lifestyle and a high-calorie diet, and appears to be associated with a set of factors that predispose to its development, including genetic factors, although these account for a small percentage of responsibility (SOUSA, 2011; CDC, 2013).

The prevalence of obesity has increased alarmingly worldwide. In 2013, it was estimated that there were around 43 million obese children under the age of 5, of which 35 million lived in developed countries and 8 million in developing countries (ONIS et al, 2010; WHO, 2014). The scenario in Europe is not much more encouraging, as it has been estimated that there are around 14 million overweight children, 3 million of whom are obese (EASO, 2013; DUARTE, 2011; DGS, 2012). It has been estimated that twenty percent of school-age children in Europe would be overweight with a high risk of developing chronic diseases when they become adults. Of these children, one in five was obese, with a significant likelihood that they were already experiencing the first signs of cardiovascular disease, diabetes and liver disease (EASO, 2013).

In the United States, there are major disparities in obesity between socio-demographic groups (WANG, 2011). According to (OGDEN, 2012), childhood obesity is becoming a national public health crisis. For a prevalence that in the periods 2003-2004 and 2009-2010, remained stable, the author reported that in 2011-2012, the prevalence of obesity in the United States was 16.9% of young people and 34.9% in adults, respectively. OGDEN also reported that in 2011-2012, 31.8% (95% CI, 29.1%-34.7%) of young Americans were overweight or obese, and 16.9% (95% CI, 14.9%-19.2%) were obese, with no statistical difference between boys and girls.

Quilombola communities are groups of individuals, whose descent is related to ethnic-racial groups, according to self-attributed criteria, with their own historical trajectory, endowed with specific territorial relations, with a presumption of black ancestry related to resistance to the historical oppression suffered. For the purposes of access to various rights, these communities are officially registered with the Palmares Cultural Foundation (BRASIL, 2009). They are population groups left over from former quilombos, representing the resistance of black Brazilians. They are located in various regions of the country, especially in rural areas, have a relative degree of geographical isolation and experience marked social and health inequalities (MONEGO, 2010).

These communities carry a great deal of historical complexity because they are the result of resistance to the process of slavery imposed for centuries on black people, who even after the Golden Law remained marginalized by society (SALLES, 2005). Many quilombos, after the abolition of slavery, gave rise to today's quilombo communities. The members of these communities have strong cultural ties, maintaining their traditions, religious practices, relationship with working the land and system of social organization (CARVALHO, 1995). From a legal point of view, quilombola communities were officially recognized by the Brazilian state in 1988, in Article 68 of the Transitional Constitutional Provisions Act (BRASIL, 2002).

The general objective of this study was to analyze the causes of childhood obesity in a quilombola community in the state of Sergipe, due to the fact that the community has no leisure and physical activity spaces, is exposed to food vulnerability and electronic habits. The specific objectives were: to verify the relationship between eating habits and obesity; to verify the relationship between physical activity and obesity; and to examine the relationship between the time spent watching television and playing video games and the presence of obesity.

II - Material and Methods

This is a cross-sectional study with a quantitative approach carried out in the quilombola community of Mussuca in the municipality of Laranjeiras/Sergipe/Brazil, selected because it is one of the largest in the state of Sergipe. The study population consisted of 301 elementary school children and adolescents aged between 5 and 14. The study ethically followed all the steps recommended by the legal instrument in force in Brazil: Resolution 466/2012(14) of the National Health Council in all phases of its execution.

The validated questionnaire (MIRANDA, 2006) was used to collect socio-demographic data and anthropometric assessment. The questionnaire consists of closed questions, which were answered by the students' guardians. This instrument was used to obtain information about the child's daily routine, physical activity and/or sports, hours spent watching television and eating habits. For the anthropometric assessment, a scale and a Leiscester stadiometer from 0 to 2 meters with its own rod were used. The students were weighed using a single measurement, standing on the scale, barefoot and wearing their uniforms, which had been weighed previously and deducted from each student's weight. Height was measured twice, with a variation of 0.5cm, with the students standing barefoot on the stadiometer platform, with their backs to the rod, feet together and in an upright position.

The time spent in physical activity was considered to be the time spent in physical education classes, sports activities, physically active leisure time and physical walking activities. Domestic activities were excluded. The time spent watching TV included only the time spent watching TV.

Students were considered obese if their body mass index (BMI) for age was equal to or greater than the 95th percentile, according to the recommendations for the cut-off point for obesity by Himes & Dietz (1994), using the BMI distribution for the Brazilian population by Anjos et al (1998).

The data was described using simple frequencies and percentages. Associations were tested using Pearson's chi-square test. The significance level adopted was 5% and the software used was R Core Team 2016.

III - Results

Of the 301 schoolchildren taking part in the study, aged between 5 and 14, enrolled in 2016 in a school in the quilombola community of Mussuca, in the municipality of Laranjeiras, state of Sergipe, northeast Brazil, 146 (49.5%) were male and 150 (50.5%) were female. These figures did not include five students who were underweight.

Table 1 shows the nutritional status (eutrophic, overweight and obese) of the number of male schoolchildren aged between 5 and 14. It can be seen that the highest percentage of overweight (25.0%) occurred at the age of 13, and the highest rate of obesity (22.2%) was at the age of 13.

Table 1 - Nutritional status of male schoolchildren from the Mussuca/Laranjeiras/SE quilombola community, by age. Quilombola community of Mussuca/Laranjeiras/SE, 2016

AGE (YEARS)	BMI			
	Eutrophic	overweight	obesity	Total
5	5(5,5%)	2(7,1%)	1(3,7%)	8(5,5%)
6	3(3,3%)	0(0,0%)	3(11,1%)	6(4,1%)
7	5(5,5%)	4(14,3%)	3(11,1%)	12(8,2%)
8	12(13,2%)	6(21,4%)	2(7,4%)	20(13,7%)
9	9(9,9%)	1(3,6%)	2(7,4%)	12(8,2%)
10	9(9,9%)	2(7,1%)	2(7,4%)	13(8,9%)
11	15(16,5%)	2(7,1%)	4(14,8%)	21(14,4%)
12	12(13,2%)	7(25,0%)	3(11,1%)	22(15,1%)
13	13(14,3%)	2(7,1%)	6(22,2%)	21(14,4%)
14	8(8,8%)	2(7,1%)	1(3,7%)	11(7,5%)
Total	**91(100,0%)**	**28(100,0%)**	**27(100,0%)**	**146(100,0%)**

Source: survey data

Table 2 shows the nutritional status (eutrophic, overweight and obese) of the number of female schoolchildren aged between 5 and 14. It can be seen that the highest percentages of overweight (25.0%) and obesity (46.2%) occurred at the age of 12.

Table 2 - Nutritional status of female schoolchildren from the Mussuca/Laranjeiras/SE quilombola community, by age. Quilombola community of Mussuca/Laranjeiras/SE, 2016

		BMI			
		eutrophic	overweight	obesity	Total
AGE (YEARS)	5	3(3,1%)	2(5,0%)	0(0,0%)	5(3,3%)
	6	3(3,1%)	3(7,5%)	0(0,0%)	6(4,0%)
	7	6(6,2%)	2(5,0%)	0(0,0%)	8(5,3%)
	8	6(6,2%)	6(15,0%)	1(7,7%)	13(8,7%)
	9	13(13,4%)	5(12,5%)	1(7,7%)	19(12,7%)
	10	8(8,2%)	5(12,5%)	0(0,0%)	13(8,7%)
	11	14(14,4%)	3(7,5%)	3(23,1%)	20(13,3%)
	12	12(12,4%)	10(25,0%)	6(46,2%)	28(18,7%)
	13	22(22,7%)	2(5,0%)	2(15,4%)	26(17,3%)
	14	10(10,3%)	2(5,0%)	0(0,0%)	12(8,0%)
Total		**97(100,0%)**	**40(100,0%)**	**13(100,0%)**	**150(100,0%)**

Source: Research data

Table 3 shows some of the eating habits of the children and adolescents. It can be seen that the majority of the participants, 188 (62.7%), ate their meals at the same time and that 256 (85%) drank soft drinks three or more times a week. These high levels of unhealthy food intake are also evident when analyzing the consumption of fast food, where 134 (44.6%) of the children and adolescents consumed this type of food two or more times a week. According to their parents, 239 (79.4%) of those surveyed were not trying to re-educate their diets.

Table 3 - Eating habits of schoolchildren from the Mussuca/Laranjeiras/SE quilombola community (N 301)

	n	%
Does your child usually eat at the same time?		
Yes	188	62,5
No	113	37,5
How many meals does your child eat during the day, including snacks?		
2 meals	15	5,0
3 meals	49	16,3
4 meals	158	52,7
Others	78	26,0
Does he/she usually eat desserts after meals?		
Yes	120	40,1
No	179	59,9
How many times a week does your child drink soft drinks?		
once	79	26,2
2 times	49	16,3
three times	125	41,5
Others	48	15,9
How many times a week does your child eat out (fast food)?		
once	167	55,5
twice	55	18,3
three times	49	16,3
Others	30	10,0
Has your child, together with the family, been trying to re-educate their diet?		
Yes	62	20,6
No	239	79,4

Source: Research data

The data shown in Table 4 shows that children and adolescents tend to be sedentary. 206 (68.4%) of these children and adolescents spent up to four hours a day in front of the television or connected to the internet, and 95 (31.6%) spent more than 5 hours a day on these activities. With regard to physical activity outside of school, 201 (66.8%) reported that they did not do so.

did any physical activity outside of school, and only 100 (33.2%) did any physical activity outside of school.

Table 4 - Screen time and physical activities of schoolchildren from the Mussuca/Laranjeiras/SE quilombola community (N 301)

	n	%
How much time per day he/she watches TV, play video games or sit at the computer?		
1 to 2 hours	66	21,9
3 to 4 hours	140	46,5
5 to 6 hours	64	21,3
More than 7 hours	31	10,3
Does your child do any physical activities outside of school?		
Yes	100	33,2
No	201	66,8
If so, which one?		
Swimming	6	6,0
Olympic Gymnastics	2	2,0
Dance	14	14,0
Other	27	27,0
Soccer	42	42,0
Handball	9	9,0

Source: Research data

Table 5 shows the relationship between BMI and the frequency of habitual consumption of certain types of food and drink and the time children and adolescents spent watching television or playing video games. It can be seen that the overweight participants (79.4%) drank soft drinks three or more times a week, while the obese mostly drank soft drinks three or more times a week (82.5%). The intake of unhealthy foods was also evident when the item fast food consumption was analyzed. Among overweight children and adolescents, 30.9%) consumed this type of food three or more times a week, while among obese people the frequency was 39.5%.

With regard to the frequency with which they watched television, video games or computers, Table 5 also shows that overweight participants (47.1%) spent more than five hours a day in front of these types of entertainment, while obese participants (60%) spent more than five hours a day in front of these devices. Among the eutrophic participants (44.7%), the overweight (10.3%) said that they did some kind of regular physical activity outside of school, while the obese (12.5%) said that they took part in some kind of physical activity.

Table 5 - BMI distribution according to the daily habits of children and adolescents (N 301), Mussuca - SE 2016.

	BMI			
	eutrophic	Overweight	obesity	X^2 (p-value)
How many times a week does your child drink soft drinks?				
once	64 (34)	8 (11,8)	5 (12,5)	71,2 (<0,001)
2 times	41 (21,8)	6 (8,8)	2 (5)	
three times	73 (38,8)	36 (52,9)	13 (32,5)	
Others	10 (5,3)	18 (26,5)	20 (50)	
How many times a week does your child eat out (fast food)?				
once	113 (60,1)	38 (55,9)	14 (35)	10,8 (0,093)
twice	34 (18,1)	9 (13,2)	10 (25)	
three times	26 (13,8)	13 (19,1)	9 (22,5)	
Others	15 (8)	8 (11,8)	7 (17,5)	
How much time per day does he/she watch TV, play video games game or is it on the computer?				
1 to 2 hours	46 (24,5)	15 (22,1)	3 (7,5)	37,4 (<0,001)
3 to 4 hours	103 (54,8)	21 (30,9)	13 (32,5)	
5 to 6 hours	26 (13,8)	24 (35,3)	14 (35)	
More than 7 hours	13 (6,9)	8 (11,8)	10 (25)	
Does your child do any physical activities outside of school?				
Yes	84 (44,7)	7 (10,3)	5 (12,5)	35,3 (<0,001)
No	104 (55,3)	61 (89,7)	35 (87,5)	
If so, which one?				
Swimming	4 (4,8)	0 (0)	2 (40)	14 (0,175)
Olympic Gymnastics	2 (2,4)	0 (0)	0 (0)	
Dance	11 (13,1)	1 (14,3)	1 (20)	
Other	24 (28,6)	2 (28,6)	0 (0)	
Soccer	35 (41,7)	4 (57,1)	1 (20)	
Handball	8 (9,5)	0 (0)	1 (20)	

Pearson's chi-square test

IV - Discussion

This study included children and adolescents, which may be a greater risk factor because they are more likely to form groups. Among 301 school children and adolescents from a quilombola community in Sergipe, aged between 5 and 14 years old, 108 (35.9%) were overweight, of which 40 (13.3%) were obese. Souza and Pinto (2007) studied quilombola children aged 9 and 10 and found that 11.7% were overweight. Guimaraes and Silva (2015) studied children aged 0 to 5 from three quilombola communities and reported the following findings: in the Santo Antônio Community, 21.4% of the children were at risk of being overweight, and (7.1%) indicated they were obese; in the África and Laranjituba Communities 64.2% of the children were eutrophic, while (21.4%), were at risk of being overweight; the Mangueiras Community had 64.7% of the children eutrophic, 11.7% were at risk of being overweight, and 11.7% were obese. Uchoa (2014) investigated the BMI of individuals in a quilombola community in Santarém/PA and found that: only 23.74% of the individuals were of ideal weight, while 19% were overweight. The author also reported that approximately 60% of the individuals were obese, with (28.6%) class one, 23.9% class two and 4.76% class three obese.

This study found a high percentage (85%) of people drinking soft drinks three times a week or more, as well as a high percentage (44.6%) of fast food snacks. According to (GRIMM, 2004), soda is a sugar-based drink with no nutritional value, which contributes to excessive consumption of empty calories. In addition, it may be replacing foods with adequate nutritional value, which contribute to the healthy growth and development of children and adolescents, such as natural juices, fruit and milk. In addition, children are the main target of indiscriminate advertising linked to sugary foods and drinks (BRASIL, 2006). FLORES, 2013, in Pelotas - RS, analyzed the consumption of soft drinks among schoolchildren from the 1st to the 4th grade, and showed that 21.6% of overweight schoolchildren drank soft drinks on a daily basis. In the quilombola community of Mussuca - Laranjeiras - SE, greater access to industrialized products and fast foods may be influenced by the location, which is very close to the state capital.

The amount of time children spend on screens or other means of electronic entertainment, and its relation to obesity, has been a frequent concern among some scholars on the subject. Uchoa (2014), in relation to the habit of watching TV, reported that individuals from the quilombola community of Santarém/PA spent more than two hours a day, on average, on this pastime. This fact, in the author's opinion, indicated a tendency to occupy themselves with an activity that required less energy, not least because the weekly time spent on physical activity was much less than the time spent using electronic devices. This study found that (47.1%) of overweight children and adolescents had an average screen time of around five hours a week, while (60%) of obese people spent more than five hours a day in front of these devices.

DE MORAES FERRARIA (2015), showed that children in the city of Sâo Caetano do Sul, in the state of Sâo Paulo are spending 500.7 min/day of sedentary time and 59.1 min/day of moderate to vigorous physical activity (MVPA), as well as 45.3% being overweight/obese. These results are similar to those of the Mussuca quilombola community, where those surveyed also showed that most children and adolescents spend more than 4 hours a day using electronic devices.

. The findings of this study showed that children and adolescents were very prone to a sedentary lifestyle. The percentage of those who regularly practiced some kind of physical activity was low. The highest percentage was among those who were eutrophic (44.7%), while among those who were obese it was only 12.5%. DE MORAES FERRARIA (2015), showed that children are spending 500.7 min/day of sedentary time and 59.1 min/day of moderate to vigorous physical activity (MVPA), in addition to 45.3% being overweight/obese. DE MAGALHÂES CARRAPEIRO, 2016, studying children aged 7 to 9 in schoolchildren in Fortaleza - CE, showed that 61.9% of schoolchildren were sedentary and that the prevalence of obesity was higher than that of overweight among overweight schoolchildren, with 55.9% (38) diagnosed with obesity and 44.1% (30) with overweight. According to JELLINGER, 2012; Sociedade Brasileira de Cardiologia, 2013) the practice of physical activity should be encouraged both by seeking a more active routine and with programmed or supervised activities. Every child or adolescent should practice at least 30 minutes of moderate-intensity activity every day. Mello et al (2004) reported that obese children tend to become sedentary, and that activity in the gym is difficult to tolerate over a long period. DIETZ, W.H. & GORTMAKER, 1985, stated that the association of obesity with some diseases, both in adults and children, has increasingly generated the need to discover its real and possible causes, in order to prevent or combat it.

According to the literature and the findings of this study, it is safe to assume that in order to burn off energy, it is not necessary to invest heavily in regular physical activity. Habits such as walking up and down stairs, skipping rope, walking to school, playing hopscotch are a great help in combating obesity, as is eating a balanced diet. Remember that diet and physical activity must be carried out simultaneously in order to prevent and treat obesity.

Conclusions

The findings of this study seem to indicate that the children and adolescents studied are at risk of overweight and obesity.

Health education based on interactive practices and dynamics with workshops for parents and students, which encourage healthy food choices, taking into account what is available to this population: juices and seasonal fruit; vegetables that could even be grown in the community, especially for the overweight and obese, who are the ones who most often use soft drinks and meals away from home.

Another point is that, as well as offering children a balanced diet and motivating them to take part in a sporting activity that gives them pleasure, we need to keep them away from a sedentary lifestyle, in an attempt to minimize the number of obese people in adulthood. Parents, the school and the physical education teacher should act as supporters of this process, as preventing childhood obesity seems to be the best way of preventing people from becoming obese adults.

The prevalence of overweight (35.9%) and obesity (13.3%) among children and adolescents in the quilombola community of Mussuca is highest at the age of 12 for girls and 13 for boys.

The higher prevalence of these health problems is associated with a higher frequency of soft drinks, eating out, screen time and not practicing physical activity.

FINAL CONSIDERATIONS

Childhood overweight is one of the main public health problems in the world, as it has a major impact on the population's morbidity pattern. Inadequate dietary intake, characterized by high consumption of simple carbohydrates and saturated fat and low consumption of fruit and vegetables, has been shown to be an important factor in the emergence of obesity.

This study suggests that food consumption plays an important role in overweight preschoolers, with excessive calorie consumption, lower fruit consumption and higher consumption of superfluous foods among the overweight group. At the same time, other variables seem to have an influence, such as early exposure to sedentary behavior and an obesogenic environment.

It is therefore suggested that school groups be given more attention, with an emphasis on prevention and treatment of individuals, in order to prevent overweight and obesity from taking hold, in other words, for the process of nutritional transition that has taken place in developed countries to take shape in Brazil.

Supervision of these children and adolescents is necessary so that constant monitoring can help with educational practices and guide the community's education and health plans.

Annex - Questionnaire (MIRANDA, 2006).

This questionnaire aims to complement the data obtained from the physical assessment that will be carried out with the children.

Beginnings of the Name: ____

1) Sex:

( ) M ( ) F

2) Age:

( ) < 20 ( ) 21 and 30( ) 31 and 40 ( ) > 40

3) At what age was your child weaned?

( ) Less than 6 months ( ) More than 1 year ( ) From 6 months to 1 year ( ) Was not breastfed

4) Do you think your child is overweight?

( ) Yes ( ) No

5) Is the family overweight in general?

( ) Yes ( ) No

6) Does your child drink water?

( ) Yes ( ) No

7) Does your child usually eat at the same time?

( ) Yes ( ) No

8) Does he/she drink liquid during meals?

( ) Yes ( ) No

9) How many meals does your child eat during the day, including snacks?

( ) 2 meals ( ) 3 meals ( ) 4 meals ( ) Other

10) Does he/she usually eat desserts after meals?

( ) Yes ( ) No

11) How many times a week does your child drink soft drinks?

( ) 1 time ( ) 2 times ( ) 3 times ( ) Other

12) How many times a week does your child eat out (fast food)?

( ) 1 time ( ) 2 times ( ) 3 times ( ) Other

13) Has your child, together with the family, been trying to re-educate their diet?

( ) Yes ( ) No

14) In your family dynamics, is it customary to reward the child with food?

( ) Yes ( ) No

15) Do your parents work outside?

( ) only the father ( ) only the mother ( ) both

16) When you both work, who do you leave your children with?

( ) alone ( ) maid ( ) grandparents ( ) Other

17) During family activities, do you often play with your child's weight?

( ) Yes ( ) No

18) Have you ever noticed your child's friends making jokes about their weight, embarrassing them or even discriminating against them?

( ) Yes ( ) No

19) Has your child suffered any recent trauma?

( ) Yes ( ) No

20) What kind of leisure activities do you do with your family at weekends?

( ) Cinema ( ) Amusement Park ( ) Other

( ) Games and sports ( ) Shopping

21) How much time a day does he/she watch TV, play video games or spend on the computer?

( ) From 1 to 2 hours ( ) From 3 to 4 hours ( ) From 5 to 6 hours ( ) More than 7 hours

22) Does your child do any physical activities outside of school?

( ) Yes ( ) No

23) If so, which

( ) Swimming ( ) Olympic Gymnastics ( ) Dance ( ) Other

( ) Football ( ) Tennis ( ) Handball

Annex I - CEP Consubstantiated Opinion

UNIVERSIDADE TIRADENTES - UNIT 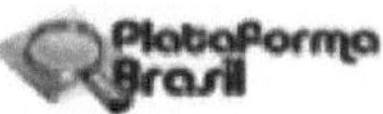

PARECER CONSUBSTANCIADO DO CEP

DADOS DO PROJETO DE PESQUISA

Título da Pesquisa: OBESIDADE INFANTO JUVENIL NA COMUNIDADE QUILOMBOLA DE MUSSUCA -
Pesquisador: LUCIANO SOUSA TEIXEIRA
Área Temática:
Versão: 2
CAAE: 57602116.6.0000.5371
Instituição Proponente: INSTITUTO DE TECNOLOGIA E PESQUISA
Patrocinador Principal: Financiamento Próprio

DADOS DO PARECER

Número do Parecer: 1.722.083

Apresentação do Projeto:
A obesidade infantil mundial vem apresentando um rápido aumento nas últimas décadas sendo caracterizada como uma verdadeira epidemia global. Este fato é bastante preocupante, pois a associação da obesidade com alterações metabólicas, como a hipertensão, e a intolerância à glicose considerados fatores de risco para o diabetes mellitus tipo 2 e as doenças cardiovasculares até alguns anos atrás eram mais evidentes em adultos, no entanto hoje já pode ser observada em crianças e adolescentes. O presente trabalho tem como objetivo avaliar a prevalência da Obesidade Infantil em grupos de crianças de sete a catorze anos da rede pública da Comunidade Quilombola de Mussuca no município de Laranjeiras no Estado de Sergipe, e identificar as suas principais causas. Para a realização deste trabalho se fez necessário a mensuração da altura e do peso de cada criança, e com base nesses dados calculou-se o IMC. Espera-se encontrar uma prevalência com valores que variam entre 5% e 18%, associação direta entre a obesidade dos pais e a obesidade dos filhos e o Sedentarismo e práticas de jogos eletrônicos.

Objetivo da Pesquisa:
Objetivo Primário:
•Determinar o perfil epidemiológico da Obesidade Infanto juvenil na Comunidade Quilombola de

Endereço: Campus Farolândia - Av. Murilo Dantas, 300 - DPE - Bloco F - Térreo
Bairro: Bairro Farolândia **CEP:** 49.032-490
UF: SE **Município:** ARACAJU
Telefone: (79)3218-2206 **Fax:** (79)3218-2100 **E-mail:** cep@unit.br

Mussuca.

Objetivo Secundário:

Identificar o percentual de crianças obesas de 06 a 14 anos nesta comunidade;

Avaliar as variáveis Antropométricas de massa corporal, estatura e peso;

Analisar o Índice de Massa Corporal (IMC).

Identificar em quais faixas etárias com maiores concentrações do problema;

Avaliação dos Riscos e Benefícios:

O projeto de pesquisa apresenta as relações de riscos e benefícios de forma adequada, de acordo com a Resolução CNS n°466/12.

Comentários e Considerações sobre a Pesquisa:

Trata-se de uma pesquisa com grande relevância científica para a área Saúde coletiva.

Considerações sobre os Termos de apresentação obrigatória:

As documentações foram inseridas corretamente e encontram-se datadas e assinadas conforme as normas descritas na Resolução CNS n° 466/12.

Conclusões ou Pendências e Lista de Inadequações:

Não há pendências ou inadequações para este projeto de pesquisa.

Considerações Finais a critério do CEP:

O CEP informa que de acordo com a Resolução CNS n° 466/12, Diretrizes e normas XI. 1 - A responsabilidade do pesquisador é indelegável e indeclinável e compreende os aspectos éticos e legais e XI. 2 - XI.2 - Cabe ao pesquisador: a) apresentar o protocolo devidamente instruído ao CEP ou à CONEP, aguardando a decisão de aprovação ética, antes de iniciar a pesquisa; b) elaborar o Termo de Consentimento Livre e Esclarecido e/ou Termo de Assentimento Livre e Esclarecido, quando necessário; c) desenvolver o projeto conforme delineado; d) elaborar e apresentar os relatórios parciais e final; e) apresentar dados solicitados pelo CEP ou pela CONEP a qualquer momento; f) manter os dados da pesquisa em arquivo, físico ou digital, sob sua guarda e responsabilidade, por um período de 5 anos após o término da pesquisa; g) encaminhar os resultados da pesquisa para publicação, com os devidos créditos aos pesquisadores associados e ao pessoal técnico integrante do projeto; e h) justificar fundamentadamente, perante o CEP ou a CONEP, interrupção do projeto ou a não publicação dos resultados.

Este parecer foi elaborado baseado nos documentos abaixo relacionados:

Endereço: Campus Farolândia - Av. Murilo Dantas, 300 - DPE - Bloco F - Térreo
Bairro: Bairro Farolândia **CEP:** 49.032-490
UF: SE **Município:** ARACAJU
Telefone: (79)3218-2206 **Fax:** (79)3218-2100 **E-mail:** cep@unit.br

Tipo Documento	Arquivo	Postagem	Autor	Situação
Informações Básicas do Projeto	PB_INFORMAÇÕES_BÁSICAS_DO_PROJETO_745700.pdf	02/09/2016 10:03:46		Aceito
Declaração de Pesquisadores	decl_de_pesquisador.pdf	23/06/2016 21:06:34	LUCIANO SOUSA TEIXEIRA	Aceito
TCLE / Termos de Assentimento / Justificativa de Ausência	TCL_.pdf	23/06/2016 21:05:55	LUCIANO SOUSA TEIXEIRA	Aceito
Declaração de Instituição e Infraestrutura	decla.pdf	23/06/2016 21:05:32	LUCIANO SOUSA TEIXEIRA	Aceito
TCLE / Termos de Assentimento / Justificativa de Ausência	tcl.pdf	23/06/2016 21:00:59	LUCIANO SOUSA TEIXEIRA	Aceito
Projeto Detalhado / Brochura Investigador	projeto_brochura.pdf	23/06/2016 20:17:06	LUCIANO SOUSA TEIXEIRA	Aceito
Folha de Rosto	folha_de_rosto.pdf	23/06/2016 20:15:56	LUCIANO SOUSA TEIXEIRA	Aceito

Situação do Parecer:
Aprovado

Necessita Apreciação da CONEP:
Não

ARACAJU, 12 de Setembro de 2016

Assinado por:
ADRIANA KARLA DE LIMA
(Coordenador)

Endereço: Campus Farolândia - Av. Murilo Dantas, 300 - DPE - Bloco F - Térreo
Bairro: Bairro Farolândia **CEP:** 49.032-490
UF: SE **Município:** ARACAJU
Telefone: (79)3218-2206 **Fax:** (79)3218-2100 **E-mail:** cep@unit.br

Annex II - Submission of article 1

ScholarOne Manuscripts

https://mc04.manuscriptcentral.com/aabcscielo

1/2

Annals of the Brazilian Academy of Sciences

Submission Confirmation □ Print

Thank you for your submission

Submitted to

Annals of the Brazilian Academy of Sciences

Manuscript ID

AABC20160744

Title

Overweight and obesity prevalence among children and adolescents in the Quilombo Community Mussuca the municipality of Laranjeiras Sergipe

Authors

Teixeira, Luciano

Date Submitted

28Oct2016

Author Dashboard

□ @ScholarOneNews | □ System Requirements | □ Privacy Statement | □ Terms of Use

□ Home

□ Author

28/10/2016 ScholarOne Manuscripts

https://mc04.manuscriptcentral.com/aabcscielo

2/

Annex III - Journal rules for submitting Article 1

Journal rules for submitting Article 1

ANNALS OF THE BRAZILIAN ACADEMY OF SCIENCES

Instructions to Authors for submitting papers

The journal ANAIS DA ACADEMIA BRASILEIRA DE CIÊNCIAS strongly encourages online submissions. Once your article has been prepared according to the instructions below, please visit the online submission site (http://aabc.abc.org.br/).

The instructions should be read carefully and followed in full. In this way, your article can be evaluated and published more efficiently and quickly. The editors reserve the right to return articles that do not comply with these instructions. Articles should be written in clear and concise English.

Objective and Editorial Policy

All articles submitted must contain original research that has not yet been published or submitted for publication. The first criterion for acceptance is scientific quality. Excessive use of abbreviations or jargon should be avoided, and articles should be understandable to as wide an audience as possible. Special attention should be paid to the Abstract, Introduction and Discussion, which should clearly draw attention to the novelty and importance of the data reported. Failure to do so could result in the article being delayed or rejected.

Texts can be published as a review, an article or as a short communication. The magazine is published quarterly in March, June, September and December.

Types of articles

Reviews: Reviews are published by invitation only. However, a review can be submitted in the form of a short letter to the Editor at any time. The letter should state the topics and authors of the proposed review and state why the subject is of particular interest to the field.

Articles: Whenever possible, articles should be subdivided into the following parts: 1. Title page; 2. Abstract (written on a separate page, 200 words or less, without abbreviations); 3. Introduction; 4. Materials and Methods; 5. Results; 6. Discussion; 7. Acknowledgements when necessary; 8. Summary and keywords (in Portuguese - foreign authors will receive assistance); 9. References. Articles in some areas, such as Mathematical Sciences, should follow their usual format. In certain cases it may be advisable to omit part (4) and combine parts (5) and (6). Where applicable, the Materials and Methods part should indicate the Ethics Committee that assessed the procedures for human studies or the standards followed for the maintenance and experimental treatment of animals.

Short communications: Short communications must be sent double-spaced. After approval, no changes to the article will be allowed, so that only typographical errors can be corrected in the proofs.

Authors should send their articles in electronic form only.

Article preparation

Articles must be prepared double-spaced. Once accepted, no changes will be made, so that only typographical errors will be corrected in the proofs.

Article length: Although articles can be as long as necessary for the concise presentation and discussion of data, succinct and carefully prepared articles are preferred both in terms of impact and ease of reading.

Tables and illustrations: Only high-quality illustrations will be accepted. All illustrations will be considered as figures, including drawings, graphs, maps, photographs and tables with more than 12 columns or more than 24 rows (maximum free figures: five figures). The probable location of the figures in the article must be indicated.

Scanned figures: Figures should be sent in accordance with the following specifications: 1. Drawings and illustrations should be in .PS/.EPS or .CDR (Postscript or Corel Draw) format and never inserted in the text; 2. Half-tone images or figures should be in .TIF format and never inserted in the text; 3. Each figure should be sent in a separate file; 4. In principle, figures should be submitted in the size in which they should appear in the journal, i.e., width of 8 cm (one column) or 12.6 cm (two columns) and with a maximum height for each figure of 22 cm or less. Figure legends must be sent double-spaced and on a separate sheet. Each linear dimension of the smallest letters and symbols must not be smaller than 2 mm after reduction. Only black and white figures will be accepted. 5) Articles on mathematics, physics or chemistry can be typed in Tex, AMS-Tex or Latex; 6) Articles without mathematical formulas can be sent in .RTF or WORD for Windows.

Title **page:** The title page should contain the following items: 1. title of the article (the title should be short, specific and informative); 2. full name(s) of the author(s); 3. professional address of each author; 4. keywords (4 to 6 words, in alphabetical order); 5. abbreviated title (up to 50 letters); 6. the name, address, fax numbers, telephone number and address of the author(s). Short title (up to 50 letters); 6. Section of the Academy to which the article belongs; 7. Name, address, fax number, telephone number and e-mail address of the author to whom all correspondence and proof of the article should be addressed.

Acknowledgements: These should be inserted at the end of the text. Personal acknowledgments should precede acknowledgments to institutions or agencies. Footnotes should be avoided; where necessary, they should be numbered. Acknowledgments of grants or scholarships, as well as acknowledgments of the collaboration of colleagues, as well as mention of the origin of an article (e.g. theses) should be indicated in this section.

Abbreviations: Abbreviations must be defined on their first occurrence in the text, except in the case of standard and official abbreviations. Units and their symbols must be in accordance with those approved by ABNT or the Bureau International des Poids et Mesures (SI).

References: Authors are responsible for the accuracy of references. Published and accepted articles (in press) can be included. Personal communications must be authorized in writing by the people involved. References to theses, abstracts from meetings, symposia (not published in indexed journals) and articles in preparation or submitted but not yet accepted may be cited in the text as (Smith et al. unpublished data) and should not be included in the list of references.

References should be cited in the text, e.g. (Smith 2004), (Smith and Wesson 2005) or, for three or more authors, (Smith et al. 2006). Two or more articles by the same author in the same year should be distinguished by letters, e.g. (Smith 2004a), (Smith 2004b) etc. Articles with three or more authors with the same first author and year of publication should also be distinguished by letters.

References should be listed in alphabetical order from the first author, always in the order of the surname XY, where X and Y are the initials. If there are more than 10 authors, use the first followed by et al. The references should have the name of the article. Journal names should be abbreviated. For the correct abbreviations, consult the database in which the journal is indexed or consult the World List of Scientific Periodicals. The abbreviation for the Annals of the Brazilian Academy of Sciences is An Acad Bras Cienc. The following examples are taken as a general guide for referencing.

Articles

Albe-Fessard D, Condes-Lara M, Sanderson P and Levante A . 1984a. Tentative explanation of the special role played by the areas of paleospinothalamic projection in patients with deafferentation pain syndromes. Adv Pain Res Ther 6: 167-182.

Albe-Fessard D, Sanderson P, Condes-Lara M, Delandsheer E, Giuffrida R and Cesaro P. 1984b. Utilization of the depression envahissante de Leâo pour l'étude de relations entre structures centrales. An Acad Bras Cienc 56: 371-383.

Knowles RG and Moncada S. 1994. Nitric oxide synthases in mammals. Biochem J 298: 249-258.

Pinto ID and Sanguinetti YT. 1984. Mesozoic Ostracode Genus Theriosynoecum Branson, 1936 and validity of related Genera. An Acad Bras Cienc 56: 207-215.

Books and book chapters

Davies M. 1947. An outline of the development of Science, Athinker's Library, n. 120. London: Watts, 214 p.

Prehn RT . 1964. Role of immunity in biology of cancer. In: National Cancer Conference , 5., Philadelphia ProceedingsPhiladelphia : J.B. Lippincott, p. 97-104.

Uytenbogaardt W and Burke EAJ . 1971. Tables for microscopic identification of minerals, 2nd ed., Amsterdam: Elsevier, 430 p.

Woody RW . 1974. Studies of theoretical circular dichroism of Polypeptides: contributions of B-turns. In: Blouts ER et al. (Eds), Peptides, polypeptides and proteins, New York: J Wiley & Sons, New York, USA, p. 338-350.

Other publications

International Kimberlite Conference , 5, 1991. Araxá, Brazil. Proceedings ... Rio de Janeiro: CPRM, 1994, 495 p.

Siatycki J . 1985. Dynamics of Classical Fields. University of Calgary, Department of Mathematics and Statistics, 19985, 55 p. Preprint n. 600.

REFERENCES

ABRANTES et al. Prevalence of overweight and obesity in children and adolescents from the Southeast and Northeast regions. J Pediatr (Rio J). 2002;78:335-40.

ABRANTES, M.M.; LAMOUNIER, J.A.; COLOSIMO, E.A. Prevalence of overweight and obesity in the Northeast and Southeast regions of Brazil. Rev. Assoc. Med. Bras., v.49, n.2, p.162-166, 2003.

ALVES, J.B.; et al. Effect of physical exercise on body weight in overweight children: randomized community clinical trial in a favela in Brazil. Cad Saude Publica.24:353-9.2008.

ALVES, J.A.B. Atividade física em crianças promovendo á saúde do adulto. Revista brasileira de saúde materno infantil;(31)1:5-6, 2003.

APCOI - Portuguese Association against Childhood Obesity (2014). "*Is obesity a problem?*" http://www.apcoi.pt/obesidade-infantil. 10-10-2015.

APN - Portuguese Association of Nutritionists (July 21, 2011). "*Obesity*". http://www.apn.org.pt/scid/webapn/defaultArticleViewOne.asp?articleID=402&categoryID= 849. 24-10-2015.

AQUINO, R.C.; PHILIPPI, S.T. Consumo infantil de alimentos industrializados e renda familiar na cidade de Sâo Paulo. Rev. Saúde Pública, v.36, n.6, p.655- 60, 2002.

BARROS, Jussara de. Educaçâo Física: Corpo em movimento available at: http://www.pedagogiaaopedaletra.com/posts/educacao-fisica-corpo-emmovimento/ accessed on September 10, 2011.

BATISTA F. M, RISSIN A. The nutritional transition in Brazil: regional and temporal trends. Cad Saude Publica. 2003;19 Suppl 1:S181-91.

BENNER,P.; et al. Educating nurses: A call for radical transformation. The Carnegie Foundation for the Advancement of Teaching, Jossey-Bass, San Francisco. 2010.

BORZEKOWSKI et al. The 30-second effect: na experiment revealing the impact of television commercials on food preferences of preschoolers. Lancet, v.37, n.9626, p.42- 6, 2001.

BRAZIL. Portal da Saúde (October 24, 2005). "*Causes and consequences of the obesity*". PortaldaSaúde : http://www.portaldasaude.pt/portal/conteudos/enciclopedia+da+saude/ministeriosaude/obesidade/causaseconsequenciasdaobesidade.htm. 20-10-2015.

BRAZIL. Decree No. 6.040, of February 7, 2007. Institutes the National Policy for the Sustainable Development of Traditional Peoples and Communities. Available at: http://www.planalto.gov.br/ccivil_03/_Ato2007-2010/2007/Decreto/D6040.htm

BRAZIL. Ministry of Education. National Institute for Educational Studies and Research (INEP). School census: 2014. Brasília, DF: MEC/INEP, 2014. Available at: Accessed on: June 21, 2015.

BRAZIL. Federal Constitution of the Republic; 1988. Transitional Constitutional Provisions Act, article 68: Ministry of Justice; 2002.

BRAZIL - Ministry of Health, National Institute of Food and Nutrition. National Health and Nutrition Survey. 2006.

BRAZIL. Special Secretariat for Policies to Promote Racial Equality. Brazil Quilombola Program. Brasília: Special Secretariat for Policies to Promote Racial Equality; 2005.

BURTON, B. T. Nutriçâo humana - manual of nutrition in health and disease. Sâo Paulo: McGraw-Hill do Brasil, 1979. 606 p

CARVALHO JJ, Doria SJ, Oliveira AN. History, tradition and struggles. Salvador: EDUFBA; 1995.

CARVALHO, Andréia Santos. Conceptions of food and nutritional security by quilombolas from the community of Tijuaçu, Bahia: an ethnographic approach to the PAA [master's degree]. **Recife: Oswaldo Cruz Foundation**, 2010.

CDC - Centers for Disease Control and Prevention (May 10, 2013). "*Public Health Genomics - Genomics and Health*". Centers for Disease Control and Prevention: http://www.cdc.gov/genomics/resources/diseases/obesity/index.htm. 25-10-2015.

CHEN, A.K.; ROBERTS,C.K.; BARNARD, R.J. Effect of a short-term diet and exercise intervention on metabolic syndrome in overweight children. Metab Clin Exp;55:871-8.2006.

COELHO, R., E BRAGANÇA, G. (2005). "Complications and Treatment of Obesity in Children". Nascer e Crescer - *Revista do Hospital de Crianças Maria Pia*, 14(2), pp. 89-91: http://repositorio.chporto.pt/bitstream/10400.16/771/1/Complica%C3%A7%C3%B5ese%2520tratamento.pdf. 28-10-2015.

COLE, T.J. et al. Establishing a standard definition for child overweight and obesity worldwide: international survey. BMJ, v.320, n.6, May, 2000. Available at www.bmj.com/cgi/content/full/320/7244/1240 Accessed April 5, 2015.

CORREA, W.; COSTA, M.A.B.; BALBINO, W. Transdisciplinary program for the sustainable development of the quilombola community of Monte Alegre. *Revista Brasileira de Pesquisa em Turismo* v. 1, n.2, p.4-53, 2007.

COUTO, C. Marketing and childhood obesity: the influence of the color of fruits and vegetables on the diet of preschool children. 2015.

CULLEN, K.; et al. Childreported family and peer influences on fruit, juice and vegetable consumption: Reliability and validity of measures. Health Education Research.;16(2):187.2001

DE CARVALHO, Helenice Aparecida; DE CARVALHO, Hêber Sebastiâo. Food & Health Project - school garden and food education at Dr. Napoleâo Sales State School - Alfenas/MG. **Extramuros-Revista de Extensâo da Univasf**, v. 2, n. 1,2014.

DE MELLO, Elza D.; LUFT, Vivian C.; MEYER, Flavia. Childhood obesity: how we can be effective. **J Pediatr (Rio J)**, v. 80, n. 3, p. 173-82, 2004.

DE SOUZA LEÂO, Leila SC. Prevalence of obesity in schoolchildren in Salvador, Bahia. **Arq Bras Endocrinol Metab**, v. 47, n. 2, 2003.

DGS - Directorate-General for Health (January 28, 2005). "*National Program to Combat Obesity*". Directorate-General for Health. Lisbon.

DGS - Directorate-General for Health (2012). "*Childhood obesity in Portugal*". Platform Against Obesity : http://www.plataformacontraaobesidade.dgs.pt/PresentationLayer/textos01.aspx?cttextoid =191&menuid=195&exmenuid=194. 22-10-2015.

DGS - Directorate-General for Health (March 31, 2013). "National Child and Youth Health Program". *Norma da Direcçâ-Geral da Saúde* n° 10/2013: http://www.dgs.pt/. 2410-2015.

DOMINGUES, Filho, Luiz Antônio. Obesity and physical activity. Jundiaí, SP: Fontoura, 2000.

DOS SANTOS, Isabela; SANTOS, Mário Jorge Silva. THE SCHOOL AND THE CONSTRUCTION OF QUILOMBOLA IDENTITY IN THE VILLAGE OF MUSSUCA/LARANJEIRAS-SE.

DUARTE, E. (2011). "*Family lifestyles and excessive weight in pre-school children*". Repository of the University of Lisbon - Doctoral Thesis: 80

EASO - European Association for the Study of Obesity (2013). "*EASO Childhood Obesity Task Force - Facts and statistics*". Retrieved November 3, 2014, from European Association for the Study of Obesity: http://easo.org/task-forces/childhood-obesity- cotf/facts-statistics.03-10-2015.

EISENBERG, Christina M. et al. Interventions to increase physical activity and healthy eating among overweight and obese children in Mexico. **salud pública de méxico**, v. 55, p. 441-446, 2013.

European Commission (May 30, 2007). White paper on a strategy for Europe on Nutrition, Overweight and Obesity related health issues. Online access: doi: http://ec.europa.eu/health/ph determinants/life style/nutrition/keydocs nutrition_en.htm

EZZATI, M. Trends in adult body-mass index in 200 countries from 1975 to 2014: a pooled analysis of 1698 population-based measurement studies with 19^2 million participants. *The Lancet,* London, v. 387, n. 10026, p. 1377- 1396, April 2, 2016.

FELDMANN, Lidiane Requia Alli et al. Psychosocial implications of childhood obesity in schoolchildren aged 7 to 12 in a mountain town in southern Brazil. **RBONE-Revista Brasileira de Obesidade, Nutriçâo e Emagrecimento**, v. 3, n. 15, 2012.

FERREIRA, H. S., M. L. D. Lamenha, A. F. S. X. Júnior, J.C. Cavalcante, and A. M. Santos. 2011. Nutrition and health of children from quilombo communities in the state of Alagoas, Brazil. *Revista Panamericana de Salud Publica* 30(1): 51-57.

FERRIANI, M.G.C.; et al. Body Self-Image of adolescents assisted in a multidisciplinary program of assistance to obese adolescents. Rev. Bras. Saúde Matern. Infant, Recife. Vol. 5. Num. 1. jan. / mar. 2005. p. 27-33.

FIATES,G.M.R.; AMBONI, R.D.M.C.; TEIXEIRA,E. Television use and food choices of children: qualitative approach. Appetite.; 50:12-8.2008.

FISBERG, M. Update on obesity in childhood and adolescence. São Paulo. Atheneu. 2005. p. 235.

FREITAS DA, Caballero AD, Marques AS, Hernández CIV, Antunes SLNO. Health and quilombola communities: a literature review. Revista CEFAC. 2011; 13: 937-43.

FULLERTON,G.; et al. Quality of life in Mexican-American children following a weight management

program. Obesity (Silver Spring).;15:2553-6.2007.
GILMAR et al. Determinants of overweight in children under 4 years of age. Jornal de Pediatría - Vol. 86, N° 4, 2010.
GIULIANO, R.; Carneiro, EC. Factors associated with obesity in schoolchildren. Jornal de Pediatria. Vol. 80. Num. 1. 2004.
GOLAN,M.; CROW,S. Parents are key players in the prevention and treatment of weight-related problems. Nutrition Reviews.;62(1):39-50.2004.
GUEDES, D.P.; et al. Prevalence of overweight and obesity in children and adolescents: estimates related to sex, age and socioeconomic class. Rev. Bras. Educ. Phys. Esp., Sao Paulo, v.20, n.3, p.151-163, 2006.
GUERRERO, A.F.H. 2010. The *Nutritional Situation of the Remaining Populations of Quilombos in the Municipality of Santarém, Pará - Brazil*. PhD Thesis, Sergio Arouca National School of Public Health, Brazil.
HALLAL, P.C.; SIMÖES, E.; REICHERT, F.F.; AZEVEDO, M.R.; RAMOS, L.R.; PRATT, M. et al. Validity and realiability of the telephone-administered international physical activity questionnaire. J Phys Act Health; 7;402-9.2010.
HENRIQUES, P. et al. Regulation of children's food advertising as a strategy for health promotion. Ciênc Saúde Colet. v.17, p.481-490, 2012.
http://www.laranjeiras.se.gov.br/historias.asp
http://www.palmares. gov.br/?page_id=88>. Accessed on January 24, 2017.
IBGE - Brazilian Institute of Geography and Statistics. **PAS - Annual Services Survey, 2012.** [online] Available on internet viaWWURL : http://www.ibge.gov.br/home/estatistica/ecnomia/comercioeservico/pas/pas2006. Archive consulted on June 11, 2013.
JANZ, K.F. et al. Sustained effect of early physical activity on body fat mass in older children. Am J Prev Med;37(1):35-40.2009.
JIANG, J. X. et al. A two-year family based behavior treatment for obese children. Archives of Disease in Childhood, 90, 1235-1238, 2005.
KOCHI, C. **Escola Saudável da Certo.** CRN-3 Magazine. News. Issue no. 76. p. 32. Dec. 2004.
LARANJEIRAS. **Black Territory:** quilombola communities. Sergipe/Laranjeiras: CELACUDE, 2006.
LEÂO, L. S. C. S.: et al. Prevalence of obesity in schoolchildren in Salvador; Bahia. **Arq. Bras. Endocrinol. Metab.** V. 47,p. 151-157, 2003.
LEITE,N.; MILANO,G.E.; CIELASK,F.; LOPES,W.A.; RODACKI,A.; RADOMINSKI, R.B. Effects of exercise and nutritional guidance on metabolic syndrome in obese adolescent. Rev Bras Fisioter.;13:73-81.2009
LUIZ, A.M.A.G.; et al. Depression, anxiety and social competence in obese children. Studies in Psychology. Vol. 10. Num. 1. 2005. p. 35-39.
MARTINS, M. T. (May 2008). "The Nurse in the Prevention of Childhood Obesity". *Sinais Vitales*, 78, 14-16.
MINISTRY OF HEALTH. National food and nutrition policy. Brasilia, 2000.
MINISTRY OF HEALTH. National food and nutrition policy. Brasilia, 2006.
MIRANDA, Tatiana C. The incidence of obesity in children from grades 1ª to 3ª in a private school in the south of São Paulo. (monograph). 2006, 57 p. Universidade Adventista de Sáo Paulo, Sáo Paulo: 2006.
MOLINA, M.C.B.; et al. Socioeconomic predictors of children's diet quality. Rev. Saúde Pública, v.44, n.5, p. s/n, 2010.
MONEGO E.T; et al. Food security of Quilombola communities in Tocantins. Seg Aliment Nutr. 2010; 17(1):37-47.
MONZAVI,R.; et al. Improvement in risk factors for metabolic syndrome and insulin resistance in overweight youth who are treated with lifestyle intervention. Pediatrics.;117:1111-8,2006.
MORENO, L. A.; RODRIGUEZ, G. Dietary risk factors for the development of childhood obesity. Current Opinion in Clinical Nutrition and Metabolic Care, 10, 336-341.2007.
MOTA, J.et al.Relationships between physical activity, obesity and meal frequency in adolescents. Annals of Human Biology, 35, 1-10, 2008.
MOURA Antonella Silva, Maria José Nobre dos Santos, Zoingridh Vieira dos Santos Faria, Jane Cláudia Jardim Pedó. Childhood obesity: a case study at the "genios educado e arte" school in the municipality of Barra dos Coqueiros/SE. V.1, n° 1 (2012).
MOREIRA, Marcella de A. et al. Overweight and associated factors in children from northeasten Brazil. **Jornal de pediatría**, v. 88, n. 4, p. 347-352, 2012.
MOREIRA, P. Overweight and obesity in Portuguese children and adolescents. **Journal of Public Health**, v.

15, n. 3, p. 155-161,2007.
MUST, Aviva; DALLAL, Gerard E.; DIETZ, William H. Reference data for obesity: 85th and 95th percentiles of body mass index (wt/ht2) and triceps skinfold thickness. **The American journal of clinical nutrition**, v. 53, n. 4, p. 839-846, 1991.
NAGLE, Brian J. et al. Interventions for the treatment of obesity among children and adolescents in Latin America: a systematic review. **salud pública de méxico**, v. 55, p. 434440, 2013.
NAHAS, M.V. et al. Physical activity, health and quality of life, concepts and suggestions for an active lifestyle.Londrina:Midiograf, 2003.
NICKLAS, T.A. et al. Impact of Commercials on Food Preferences of Low-income, Minority Preschoolers. J Nutr Educ Behav, v.43, p. 35 - 41, 2010.
NORGREN, R. et al. Gustatory reward and the nucleus accumbens. *Physiol. Behav.*,v.89, n.4, p.531-5, 2006.
NUNES, SUSANA. (2008). "*Adipocyte Rebound in Childhood and the Prediction of Obesity*". University of Porto. Faculty of Nutrition and Food Sciences. Monograph.
OGDEN, C. et al. Prevalence of childhood and adult obesity in the United States, 20112012. **Jama**, v. 311, n. 8, p. 806-814, 2014.
WHO (World Health Organization). Obesity: preventing and controlling the global epidemic - WHO consultancy report, São Paulo: Roca, 2004.
ONIS, et al. (2010). "Global prevalence and trends of overweight and obesity among preschool children". *American Journal of Clinical Nutrition*. 92, pp. 1257-1264:
OPPERMAN, C. S., and CASSANDRA, K. A. (2001). "*Pediatric Nursing Contemporânea*". Loures: Lusociência.
PATRICK,H.; NICKLAS,T. The benefits of authoritative feeding style: caregiver feeding styles and children's food consumption patterns. Appetite, 44, 243-249, 2005.
PELLANDA LC. et al. Ischemic disease: prevention begins during childhood. J. Pediatr, Rio de Janeiro, 2002; 78(2):91-96.
POETA,L.S.; et al. Interdisciplinary intervention in obese children and impact on health and quality of life. J Pediatr (Rio J); 89:499-504, 2013.
PEREIRA, A. L. School food policy for specific populations: Quilombolas. Available at: <http://www.rebrae.com.br>. Accessed on: May 7, 2009.
PINTO A.R; et al. Quilombos do Brasil: Segurança Alimentar e Nutricional em territórios titulados. V. 20. Brasília, DF: Ministério do Desenvolvimento Social e Combate à Fome; Secretaria de Avaliaçâo e Gestâo da Informaçâo; 2014.
POLLOCK, M.L. et al. **Exercise in Health and Disease. Assessment and Prescription for Prevention and Rehabilitation.** 1. ed. Rio de Janeiro: Editora Médica e Científica, 1986.
REGO, et al (2007). "*Growing up - How to prevent or treat obesity in children and adolescents*". Lisbon: Works in progress.
RÊGO, C. (2010). "Influence of early nutritional experiences on the genesis of adult diseases". *Revista Factores de Risco*. 21, pp. 34-41.
REZENDE, Adriana Arruda Barbosa et al. CARDIOVASCULAR RISK FACTORS IN CHILDREN FROM A PUBLIC SCHOOL IN THE MUNICIPALITY OF GURUPI- TO. **AMAZÔNIA: SCIENCE & HEALTH**, v. 2, n. 4, p. 2 a 8, 2014.
RIBEIRO, S. F. (August 2008). " *Childhood Obesity'.* ubithesis: https://ubithesis.ubi.pt/handle/10400.6Z851. 23-10-2015
RIBEIRO, Graciele; DE OLIVEIRA MORAIS, Franciny Michelle; DE PINHO, Lucinéia. (In) Food security of quilombola community in the north of Minas Gerais/Food (in) security of quilombola community in the north of Minas Gerais. **Ciencia, Cuidado e Saude,** v. 14, n. 3, p. 1245-1250, 2015.
RITO, Ana. Nutritional status of children and pre-school food supply in the municipality of Coimbra, Portugal, 2001. **Rio de Janeiro: Sérgio Arouca National School of Public Health**, 2004.
SALLES, V. 2005. *The Negro in Pará under Slavery*. Belém: IAP.
SANTOS, L. A.S., et al. National school feeding program in the context of municipalization. In: Sandra Maria Chaves (Org.) Avaliaçâo de Políticas de Segurança Alimentar e Nutriçâo no Estado da Bahia. Sâo Paulo-SP: Prol Editora Gráfica, 2008, v. 2, p. 185-226.
SATO,Y.; et al. Clinical aspects of physical exercise for diabetes/metabolic syndrome. Diabetes Res Clin Pract Suppl.;77:87-91, 2007.
SAWAYA, Ana Lydia; FILGUEIRAS, Andrea. "Open happiness"? Implications for food addiction. **Estudos Avançados**, v. 27, n. 78, p. 53-70, 2013.

SHAMAH-LEVY T, Villalpando-Hernández S, Rivera-Dommarco JA. Nutrition results from ENSANUT 2006. Cuernavaca, Mexico: National Institute of Public Health, 2007.

SHI, L.; MAO, Y. Excessive recreational computer use and food consumption behavior among adolescents. Ital J Pediatr, v.36, n.1, p. 1- 4, 2010.

SILVA, D. O.; et al. de. The causal network of food and nutritional insecurity in a quilombola community with the construction of the BR 163 highway, Pará, Brazil. Revista de Nutriçâo da Puccamp, Campinas, 21(suplemento), p. 83s-97s, jul./ago. 2008.

SOARES, L. D., and PETROSKI, E. L. (2003). "Prevalence, Etiologic Factors and Treatment of Childhood Obesity". *Revista Brasileira de Cineantropometria e Desempenho Humano*, 5(1), pp. 63-74: http://150.162.1.115/index.php/rbcdh/article/view/4008/3405. 28-09-2015.

SOUSA, J. (2011). "*Childhood Obesity in Portugal - Association with Eating Habits, Physical Activity and Sedentary Behaviors of School-aged Adolescents in Mainland Portugal*". Lisbon: Colibri.

TADDEI, J. **Nutritional deviations in children under five years of age: evidence from national anthropometric surveys [Thesis].** Sâo Paulo: Paulista School of Medicine, Federal University of Sâo Paulo, 2000.

TENORIO, M.C.M.; et al. Physical activity and sedentary behavior in adolescent high school students. Ver Bras Epidemiol;13:105-17, 2010.

TOEWS, et al (2004). "*Feeding our children - A guide to happy and healthy growth*". Lisbon: Livros Horizonte.

VETRINI, N. Maternal feeding styles of overweight and normal weight mothers as predictors of child weight status and energy intake. United States -- New Jersey: Rutgers The State University of New Jersey - New Brunswick; 2009.

VIGITEL. Vigitel Brazil 2014: Surveillance of risk and protective factors for chronic diseases by telephone survey. Ministério da Saúde (MS), Secretaria de Vigilancia em Saúde, Secretaria de Gestao Estratégica e Participativa. Brasilia: MS; 2014.

YEOMANS, M. R. Taste, palatability and the control of appetite. *Proc. Nutr. Soc.*, v.57,n.4, p.609-15, 1998.

WANG, Y. Disparities in pediatric obesity in the United States. **Advances in Nutrition: An International Review Journal**, v. 2, n. 1, p. 23-31, 2011.

WORLD HEALTH ORGANIZATION - Obesity preventing and managing the Global Epidemic: Report of a WHO Consulation of Obesity. Geneva, WHO/NUT/NCD, 1998

WORD HEALTH ORGANIZATION. Report of a WHO Consulation on Obesity. Preventing and managing the global epidemic. **WHO,** Geneve, 1998.

WHO - World Health Organization (2014). "*Obesity and overweight".* World Health Organization: http://www.who.int/mediacentre/factsheets/fs311/en/ 24-10-2015.

APN - Portuguese Association of Nutritionists (July 21, 2011). "Obesity. http://www.apn.org.pt/scid/webapn/d efaultArticleViewOne.asp?articleID= 402&categoryID=849. 24/10/2015.

Brazil. Federal Constitution; Act 1988. Constitutional Provisions, Article 68: Ministry of Justice; 2002.

Carvalho, Andreia Santos. Conceptions of food and nutrition security for the Maroons Tijua^u community, Bahia: an ethnographic approach to the PAA [master]. Recife: Oswaldo Cruz Foundation, 2010.

Carvalho JJ, Doria SJ, Oliveira AN. History, tradition and struggles. Salvador: EDUFBA; 1995.

DGS - Directorate General for Health (March 31, 2013)... "National Child Health Program and Youth". Standard of Health DirectorateGeneralNo . 10/2013: http://www.dgs.pt/. 24/10/2015.

DGS - Directorate General of Health (2012). "The Child obesity in Portugal." Platform Against Obesity: http://www.plataformacontraaobesidade.dgs.pt/PresentationLayer/textos 01.aspx?cttextoid=191&menuid=195 &exmenuid=194. 22/10/2015.

CDC - Centers for Disease Control and Prevention (May 10, 2013). "Public Health Genomics - Genomics and Health". Centers for Disease Control and Prevention : http://www.cdc.gov/genomics/resour ces/diseases/obesity/index.htm. 25/10/2015.

Duarte, E. (2011). "Family lifestyles and excessive weight gain in children of preschool age." Repository of the University of Lisbon - PhD thesis: 80

EASO - European Association for the Study of Obesity (2013). "EASO Childhood Obesity Task Force - Facts and statistics". Retrieved on November 3, 2014, the European Association for the Study of Obesity: http://easo.org/task- forces/childhood-obesity-cotf/facts- statistics.03-10-2015.

Eisenberg, Christina M. et al. Interventions to Increase physical activity and healthy eating Among overweight

and obese children in Mexico. salud pública mexico, v. 55, p. 441-446, 2013.
Ferreira, Haroldo da Silva et al. Nutrition and health of children of the remaining communities of quilombos in the state of Alagoas, Brazil. 2011.
Gilmar et al. determinants of overweight factors in children under 4 years of age. Jornal de Pediatria - Vol 86, No. 4, 2010.
Guerrero, A.F.H. 2010. Nutritional SituationQuilomboRemnant
populations of the municipality of Santarém, Pará - Brazil. Doctoral Thesis, National School of Public Health Sergio Arouca, Brazil.
Lima, Severina Carla Vieira Cunha et al. the usualdiet of childrenand adolescentswith overweight and
obesity evaluation. Campinas: Journal of Nutrition 2004.
Mello, E. D. et al. Childhood obesity: how can we be effective? Sao Paulo: Brazilian Society of Pediatrics: Journal of Pediatrics 2004.
Miranda, Tatiana C. The incidence of obesity in children from 1st to 3rd grade in a private school in the south of Sáo Paulo. (monograph). 2006 57 p. Adventist University of Sáo Paulo, Sáo Paulo: 2006.
Monego E.T, Peixoto MRG, Lamb MM, RM Costa. food security of Tocantins Quilombo communities. Mon Aliment Nutr. 2010; 17 (1): 37-47.
Moura, Antonella Silva, Maria José Nobre dos Santos, Zoingridh Vieira dos Santos Faria, Jane Claudia Pedó Garden. Childhood Obesity: a case study in school "geniuses education and art" the municipality of Barra dos Coqueiros / SE. V.1, No. 1 (2012).
Nagle, Brian J. et al. Interventions for the treatment of obesity Among children and adolescents in Latin America: a systematic review. salud pública mexico, v. 55, p. 434-440, 2013.
OGDEN, C. et al. Prevalence of childhood and adult obesity in the United States, 2011-2012. Jama v. 311, no. 8, p. 806-814, 2014.
ONIS, et al. (2010). "Global prevalence and trends of overweight and obesity Amongpreschoolchildren ".
American Journal of Clinical Nutrition. 92, pp. 1257-1264:
Ribeiro, S. F. (August 2008). "Child obesity". ubithesis:
https://ubithesis.ubi.pt/handle/10400. 6/851. 10/23/2015
Salles, V. 2005. *The Black Man in Para Under Slavery*. Belem: IAP.
Souza, Elaine Avila Cunha. Prevalence of Obesity in Children and Adolescents in School of the Municipal Taubate Elaine Avila Souza Cunha, Aline Llanos de Oliveira 2, Francisco Santos Pinto Filho 3, Ana Lourdes Correa 4.
Sousa, J. (2011). "Obesity Children and Youth in Portugal - Association with Eating Habits, Physical Activity and Sedentary Behaviors of Adolescents Portugal Continental Schooled". Lisbon: Colibri.
Toews, et al (2004). "The Power of our children - Guide to a happy and healthy growth." Lisbon: Books
Horizon.
Uchoa, Jackson Nogueira et al. Nutritional profile of lowland areas of communities and quilombolas plateau and its relationship with hypertriglyceridemia
HYPERCHOLESTEROLEMIA, IN SANTAREM-PA MUNICIPALITY. Magazine FOCUS-Hope Foundation / IESPES, v. 1, no. 22, p. 14-19, 2014.

Wang, Y. Disparities in pediatric obesity in the United States.**Advances in Nutrition: An International Review Journal**, v. 2, n. 1, p. 23-31, 2011
WHO - World Health Organization *(2014). "Obesity and overweight".*
WorldHealthOrganization :
http://www.who.int/mediacentre/facts heets/fs311/en/ 24-10-2015.
WHO - World Health Organization *(2014). "Obesity and overweight".*
WorldHealthOrganization :
http://www.who.int/mediacentre/facts heets/fs311/en/ 24-10-20
ANJOS L.A, Veiga GV, Castro IRR. Distribution of body mass index values in the Brazilian population up to 25 years of age. **Panam Salud Publica 1998**;3(3): 164-73.
APN - Portuguese Association of Nutritionists (July 21, 2011). "*Obesity*". http://www.apn.org.pt/scid/webapn/defaultArticleViewOne.asp?articleID=402&categoryID=84 9. 24-10-2015.
BRAZIL. Ministry of Health. Health Care Secretariat. Department of Basic Care. Obesity. Brasilia: The

Ministry; 2006. [Caderno de Aten^áo Básica n° 12. Série A. Normas e Manuais Técnicos].
BRAZIL. Federal Constitution of the Republic; 1988. Ato das Disposi^óes Constitucionais Transitórias, artigo 68: Ministério da Justina; 2002.
BRAZIL. National Education Development Fund. Resolution/FNDE/CD/No 38, of July 16, 2009. Provides for school meals and the Money Directly at School Program for basic education students and other measures. *Diário Oficial da Uniao* 2009; July 17, 2009.
CARVALHO JJ, Doria SJ, Oliveira AN. History, tradition and struggles. Salvador: EDUFBA; 1995.
CDC - Centers for Disease Control and Prevention (May 10, 2013). "*Public Health Genomics - Genomics and Health*". Centers for Disease Control and Prevention: http://www.cdc.gov/genomics/resources/diseases/obesity/index.htm. 25-10-2015.
DE MAGALHÁES CARRAPEIRO, Mariana. Relationship between obesity and eating behavior and lifestyle in Brazilian schoolchildren. 2016
DE MORAES FERRARIA, Gerson Luis et al. Association between electronic equipment in the bedroom and sedentary lifestyle, physical activity, and body mass index of children. 2015.
DIETZ, W.H. & GORTMAKER, S.L. Do we fatten our children at the television set? Obesity and television viewingin children and adolescents. Pediatrics. 1985; 75(5): 807- 812.
DGS - Diredo-Geral da Saúde (2012). '*Childhood obesity in Portugal'.* Platform Against Obesity : http://www.plataformacontraaobesidade.dgs.pt/PresentationLayer/textos01.aspx?cttextoid=1 91&menuid=195&exmenuid=194. 22-10-2015.
DGS - Diredo-Geral da Saúde (March 31, 2013). "National Child and Youth Health Program". *Norma da Direcqa-Geral da Saúde* n° 10/2013: http://www.dgs.pt/. 24-10-2015.
DUARTE, E. (2011). "*Family lifestyles and excessive weight in pre-school children*". Repository of the University of Lisbon - Doctoral Thesis: 80
EASO - European Association for the Study of Obesity (2013). "*EASO Childhood Obesity Task Force - Facts and statistics*". Retrieved November 3, 2014, from European Association for the Study of Obesity: http://easo.org/task-forces/childhood-obesity-cotf/facts- statistics.03-10-2015.
FLORES, Thayná Ramos et al. Consumption of soft drinks among primary school students in the city of Pelotas, Rio Grande do Sul. **Ciencia & Saúde**, v. 6, n. 1, p. 59-66, 2013.
GRIMM GC, Harnack L, Story M. Factors associated with soft drink consumption in schoolaged children. J Am Diet Assoc, 2004; 104(8):1244-9.
GUIMARÂES, R. C. R.; SILVA, H. P. Nutritional status and growth of quilombola children from different communities in the state of Pará. **Amazônica-Revista de Antropología**, v. 7, n. 1, p. 186-209, 2015.
HIMES JH, Dietz WH. Guidelines for overweight in adolescent preventive services recommendations from an Expert Committee. **Am J Clin Nutr 1994**;59:307-16.
JELLINGER PS, Smith DA, Mehta AE, Ganda O, Handelsman Y, Rodbard HW, et al. American Association of Clinical Endocrinologists' Guidelines for Management of Dyslipidemia and Prevention of Atherosclerosis. Endocr Pract, 2012;18 (Suppl 1):1-78.
KNITTLE, J.L. et al. The growth of adipose tissue in children and adolescents. Journal of Clinical Investigation. 1979; 63(2): 239-246.
MALINA, R.M. & BOUCHARD, C. Growth, Maturation and Physical Activity. Champaign: Human Kinetics Books, 1991.
MELLO, Elza D. de et al. **Childhood obesity: how can we be effective?** Sao Paulo: Brazilian Society of Pediatrics: Journal of Pediatrics: 2004.
MIRANDA, Tatiana C. The incidence of obesity in children from 1ª to 3ª grades in a private school in the south of Sao Paulo. (monograph). 2006, 57 p. Universidade Adventista de Sao Paulo, Sao Paulo: 2006.
MONEGO ET, Peixoto MRG, Cordeiro MM, Costa RM. Food security in Quilombola communities in Tocantins. Seg Aliment Nutr. 2010; 17(1):37-47.
OGDEN, C. et al. Prevalence of childhood and adult obesity in the United States, 20112012. **Jama**, v. 311, n. 8, p. 806-814, 2014.
OLIVEIRA, Cecília L. de and FISBERG, Mauro. **Obesity in childhood and adolescence**: **a real epidemic**. *Arq Bras Endocrinol Metab* [online]. 2003, vol.47, n.2, pp. 107-108. ISSN 0004-2730.
ONIS, et al. (2010). "Global prevalence and trends of overweight and obesity among preschool children". *American Journal of Clinical Nutrition.* 92, pp. 1257-1264:
RIBEIRO, S. F. (August 2008). " *ObesidadeInfantil*". ubithesis: https://ubithesis.ubi.Pt/handle/10400.6/851. 23-10-2015
RIBEIRO, J. L. P. (1999). *Investigaçao e avaliaçao em Psicología da Saúde*. Lisbon: Climepsi Editores.

SALLES, V. 2005. *The Negro in Pará Under Slavery*. Belém: IAP.
SOUZA, Elaine Cristina de Ávila Cunha. Prevalence of Obesity in Children and Adolescents at a Municipal School in Taubaté Elaine Cristina de Ávila Cunha Souza, Aline Llanos de Oliveira 2, Francisco Santos Pinto Filho 3, Ana de Lourdes Correa 4.
Brazilian Society of Cardiology. Arquivos brasileiros de cardiologia, 2013; 101(6): 28-30.
SOUSA, J. (2011). "*Childhood Obesity in Portugal - Association with Eating Habits, Physical Activity and Sedentary Behaviors of School-aged Adolescents in Mainland Portugal*". Lisbon: Colibri.
UCHOA, Jackson Nogueira et al. THE NUTRITIONAL PROFILE OF QUILOMBOLAS FROM COMMUNITIES IN THE VARIETY AND PLANALTO AREAS AND ITS RELATIONSHIP WITH HYPERTRIGLYCERIDEMIA AND HYPERCHOLESTEROLEMIA IN THE MUNICIPALITY OF SANTARÉM.
PA. **Revista EM FOCO-Fundagao Esperanga/IESPES**, v. 1, n. 22, p. 14-19, 2014
WANG, Y. Disparities in pediatric obesity in the United States.**Advances in Nutrition: An International Review Journal**, v. 2, n. 1, p. 23-31, 2011
WHO - World Health Organization. Report of a WHO Consultation on Obesity. **Preventing and managing the global epidemic.** WHO, Geneve, **1998**.
WHO - World Health Organization (2014). "*Obesity and overweight*". World Health Organization: http://www.who.int/mediacentre/factsheets/fs311/en/ 24-10-2015.

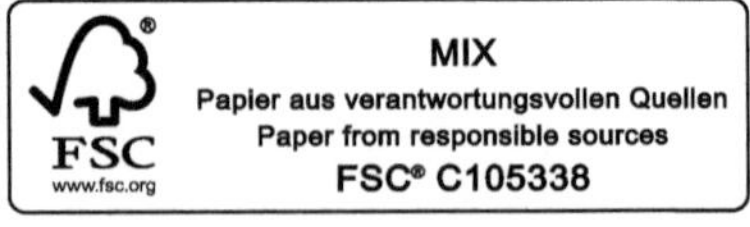

Printed by Books on Demand GmbH, Norderstedt / Germany